LEICESTER POLYTECHNIC LIBRARY
CITY CAMPUS
Telephone 551551

Please return this book on or before the last date stamped
below.

Fines will be charged on books returned after this date.

18/7/01 Ave R570

- 6 DEC 2011

14.	2 3 FEB 1999	
	3 1 OCT 2001	
26. JUN. 1993	1 4 JUN 2002	
21. APR 94	1 3 JUN 2003	
24. FEB 95	1 OCT 2004	
17. MAR 85	2 7 FEB 2005	
24. NOV	2 9 OCT 2007	
2 0 JUN 1997	15th Nov 2007	

Synthetic Biomedical Polymers
Concepts and Applications

Edited by: M. Szycher and W.J. Robinson

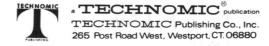

a TECHNOMIC® publication
TECHNOMIC Publishing Co., Inc.
265 Post Road West, Westport, CT. 06880

Synthetic Biomedical Polymers
Concepts and Applications

Edited by: M. Szycher and W.J. Robinson

a TECHNOMIC publication

Copyright 1980 TECHNOMIC Publishing Company, Inc.
265 Post Road West, Westport, CT. 06880

Printed in U.S.A.
Library of Congress Card No. 80-52137
ISBN 087762-290-6

This book is dedicated to our wives,
Laurie and Mary

for constant support, inspiration and patience.

Synthetic Biomedical Polymers:
Concepts & Applications

Contributing Authors

Beach William, F., Ph.D.
Group Leader
Union Carbide Corporation
Chemicals & Plastics Division
One River Road
Bound Brook, New Jersey 08805
(201) 356-8000

Bonk, Henry W., BS
Manager, Elastomers
The Upjohn Company
Donald S. Gilmore Research Laboratories
North Haven, Connecticut 06463
(203) 281-2700

Boretos, John W., Ph.D.
Biomedical Engineering and Instrumentation Branch
Division of Research Services
National Institutes of Health
Bethesda, Maryland 20014

Colovos, George C., BS,MS
The Upjohn Company
Donald S. Gilmore Research Labs
North Haven, Connecticut 06473
(203) 281-2700

Daly, Benedict, D.T., M.D.
Department of Cardiothoracic Surgery
Tufts New England Medical Center
and St. Elizabeth's Hospital
Boston, MA

Donachy, James H., Research Associate; Dept. of Surgery
Fabrication Specialist
The Pennsylvania State University
312 Mechanical Engineering
University Park, Pennsylvania 16802
(717) 534-8328

Hillegass, Donald V.
Research Chemist, Research Division
Goodyear Tire and Rubber Co.
Akron, Ohio
(216) 794-2124

Hoffman, Allan S., D.Sc.
Professor
Department of Chemical Engineering
and Center for Bioengineering
University of Washington
Seattle, Washington 98195

Hodge, J.W. Jr., Ph.D.
General Engineer
US Army Medical Bioengineering Research
  and Development Laboratory
Fort Detrick
Frederick, Maryland 21701 (301) 663-7237

Kiraly, Raymond J., MS, ME
Director of Engineering
Department of Artificial Organs
Cleveland Clinic Foundation
Cleveland, Ohio
(216) 444-2470

Kronick, Paul L., Ph.D.
The Franklin Institute Research Laboratories
Philadelphia, PA 19103

Phillips, Winfred, M., D.Sc.
Professor
College of Engineering
The Pennsylvania State University
312 Mechanical Engineering
University Park, Pennsylvania 16802

Pierce, William S., M.D.
Professor
College of Medicine
The Pennsylvania State University
312 Mechanical Engineering
University Park, Pennsylvania 16802

Poirier, Victor L., BS,ME
Manager, Biomedical Division
Thermo Electron Corporation
Research and Development Center
Biomedical Systems Department
45 First Avenue
Waltham, MA 02154

Ratner, Buddy, D., Ph.D.
Department of Chemical Engineering and
Center for Bioengineering
University of Washington
Seattle, Washington 98195

Refojo, Miguel, F., D.Sc.
Eye Research Institute of Retina Foundation
and Department of Ophthalmology
Harvard Medical School
Boston, MA

Robinson, William J., BSEE
Thermo Electron Corporation
Research and Development Center
Waltham, MA 02154

Rosenberg, Gerson, Ph.D.
Senior Project Associate
College of Medicine
The Pennsylvania State University
312 Mechanical Engineering
University Park, Pennsylvania 16802

Szycher, Michael, BS Chem Eng, MA Cardiac Phys
Thermo Electron Corporation
Research and Development Center
Biomedical Systems Department
45 First Avenue
Waltham, MA 02154

F.R. Tittmann
Development Scientist
Union Carbide Corporation
Chemicals & Plastics Division
One River Road
Bound Brook, New Jersey 08805
(201) 356-8000

Ulrich, Henry, Ph.D.
The Upjohn Company
Donald S. Gilmore Research Laboratories
North Haven, Connecticut 06473

Wade, C.W.R., Ph.D.
Research Chemist
US Army Medical Bioengineering Research and
    Development Laboratory
Fort Detrick
Frederick, Maryland 21702

Table of Contents

A Special Message to the Readers of
Synthetic Biomedical Polymers
from the authors

The field of Synthetic Biomedical Polymers is relatively new and, as such, not yet sharply defined. Undoubtedly, a thorough understanding of synthetic polymer chemistry is an obligatory requirement; but what about the "biomedical" qualifier? It is apparent that some background in the classical life sciences (anatomy, physiology, biochemistry and biophysics) is also important. Therefore, the approach taken in this book is multi-disciplinary: the reader will quickly discern that polymer chemistry is only a foundation, being reinforced by plastic engineering, histology, hematology, anatomy and other disciplines too numerous to mention.

Before undertaking the book, we deliberated over what subject matter was most appropriate, what value it could provide, and who could benefit. A careful review of the existing literature revealed that there are several good texts on the subject, and that specialized journals cover a multitude of subjects. The literature also points out that there has been a transition from the pragmatism or serendipity of early investigators, into a more controlled, goal-oriented approach. Earlier attempts concentrated in selecting commercially available polymers, cleaning or purifying them as much as possible, and using them as the starting points in the fabrication of prototype prostheses. Lately, the tendency has been to synthesize those polymers most suitable to the intended application, polymers so specialized that they may never become commercially viable, except for their use in biomedical applications.

With these thoughts in mind, the intent of this text is to emphasize, from a practical approach, the chemical and physical aspects of synthesis and fabrication as well as the properties of those polymers which are most compatible with biologic organisms. The approach has been to cover as many applications of synthetic biomedical polymers as possible and at the same time examine as many stages of their development as possible. The result is that we have cut across disciplines, centers of research, and topics in an effort to present a broad view of the field. The subject matter should be of interest to uninitiated as well as experienced polymer chemists, physical and biological scientists, physicians, surgeons, and engineers.

Development in the field is a dynamic state where new findings are constantly emerging. We have not covered all of the field or developments, nor have we limited the emphasis to a given area. Two families of polymers, however, are highlighted — polyurethanes and hydrogels — since they have proven to be highly compatible with living systems, as well as being suitable to multiple fabrication methods and end products.

The contributors in this book represent the various disciplines cited previously and the topics originate from investigations conducted in the private and government as well as academic sectors. Some of the most fruitful applications of synthetic polymers are found in artificial heart research and development: this is reflected in the first eight chapters, which present diverse approaches to blood contacting surfaces and delineate the chemical and physical requirements of the various materials. Hydrogens, as a family, are promising materials for biomedical applications: three chapters describe hydrogels that use radiation curing as well as the more controversial aqueous phase during methods. The last three chapters discuss fresh approaches to long standing problem areas in prosthesis development.

This book would not have been possible without the efforts of the contributors, who represent the vanguard of this young emerging field. The interest of the Society of Plastics Engineers and the support of Thermo Electron Corporation cannot be understated. Specifically, we would like to acknowledge the support and cooperation of these people who have been there on a daily basis: John T. Keiser, Vice President, Research and Development Center/New Business Division, and Victor L. Poirier, Manager, Biomedical Systems, our mentors; Dorothy L. Carchia and Thomas L. Coyne, editorial and graphic assistance; and Claudia W. Chase, communications and manuscripts.

Waltham, Massachusetts

Michael Szycher
William J. Robinson

AN INTEGRATED APPROACH TO HEMOCOMPATIBLE POLYMERS: A TEST PROTOCOL

Michael Szycher

Thermo Electron Corporation
Research and Development Center
Biomedical Systems Department
45 First Avenue
Waltham, Massachusetts 02154

ABSTRACT

The successful design and fabrication of bladders intended for use in cardiac assist devices demands the identification, synthesis, and successful selection of hemocompatible polymers possessing long-term flexure endurance, and chemical stability when exposed to the degrading effects of the biological environment. A test matrix has been evolved at Thermo Electron that represents an integrated, multidisciplinary approach to ascertain whether a candidate biomaterial fulfills these needs. Our protocol involves a multifaceted test matrix capable of predicting long-term behavior of polymers. The tests include relevant, complementary assays performed in vitro under simulated physiologic conditions, as well as in vivo tests involving laboratory animals.

This chapter presents a matrix of mechanical, physical, and chemical tests to assay certain properties of candidate biomaterials that are relevant to their long-term performance and reliability. The objective of this test procedure is to use acquired data to predict the overall usefulness of candidate polymers for possible use as hemocompatible prosthetic devices. The essence of this procedure is the systematic delineation of test protocols and methodology designed to predict long-term biomaterials performance.

The test matrix attempts to correlate the general mechanical behavior of polymers to both environmental and structural factors. Environmental factors include exposure to physiological fluids, time, and cyclic loading. Structural factors include molecular weight, branching, crosslinking, copolymerization, and crystalline morphology. This protocol has been utilized at the Biomaterials Laboratories of Thermo Electron Corporation to assist in the collection of relevant and timely data in our search for durable, functional, and biologically stable materials.

MATERIALS EVALUATION SCHEMA

The evaluation of candidate biomaterials is based on a matrix protocol that follows a step-by-step approach. The effort is divided into segmented steps, performed concurrently, each a logical sequel to its predecessor. (Table 1, Figure 1).

Table 1. Test Matrix Summary

Test Group	Method	Response
Chemical Assessments	Hydrolytic Stability Oxidative Stability Infrared Spectroscopy Attenuated Total Reflectance Gel Permeation Chromatography Differential Scanning Calorimetry	Possible Degradation Chemical Group Identification Surface Chemical Group Identification Molecular Weight Distribution Measurement of: Transitions, Purity, Cure
Physical Chemical Analyses	Solution Rheology Intrinsic Viscosity	Molecular Weight Determination
Mechanical Properties	Stress/Strain Properties Viscoelastic Properties Mock Loop Testing on Prototypes	Ultimate Polymer Strength Measurement of Transitions, Viscoelastic Flow, Damping Coefficient Real-Time Fatigue Testing
Biological	In Vitro and Ex Vivo	Acute Biocompatibility

DATA ACQUISITION PROTOCOL

Chemical Assessments

In general, biomedical polymers can be divided into two major groups — those used as flexible prostheses, and those intended for rigid applications. Cardiovascular prostheses, and those intended for rigid applica-

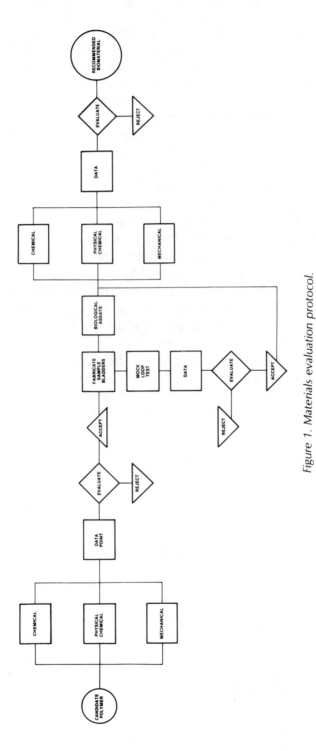

Figure 1. Materials evaluation protocol.

tions. Cardiovascular prostheses are often soft and flexible; therefore, polymers designed to transport or pump blood must meet a more stringent set of qualifications. In addition to passing obvious requirements of blood compatibility and stability, these polymers must also remain flexible and elastic over extensive periods of time.

To accurately determine which candidate polymers are capable of meeting the high standards necessary for biomedical applications, a thorough understanding of polymer degradation mechanisms is essential. Macromolecules are susceptible to various modes of degradation; chemically induced degradation includes thermal, oxidative, hydrolytic, and perhaps biological. In addition to these, polymers under constant flexing are susceptible to fatigue (mechanical decay).

Thermal degradation generall occurs by heat-induced chain scission, with subsequent depolymerization. *Oxidation* can be initiated through the coupling of free oxygen with a chemical compound, followed by molecular decomposition into reactive radicals. The radicals then attach primary chemical bonds, eventually leading to chain scission and depolymerization. *Biological* degradation could occur by the cleavage of polymer chains under the influence of enzymes. *Hydrolysis* generally occurs in polyester-based polyurethanes, when the polymer is exposed to an aqueous environment for prolonged periods; since the biological environment is aqueous, polyurethane elastomers intended as biomedical prostheses should be thoroughly tested to ensure being hydrolytically stable.

Our test matrix is thus divided into four groups: chemical, physicochemical, mechanical, and biological. A brief description of the tests follows.

Hydrolytic Stability

If macromolecules lose their physical integrity when exposed to an aqueous environment, the major degradation mechanism is usually hydrolysis. Since it is of the utmost importance that polymers remain unchanged when implanted within a living body, a crucial first step is to ascertain the hydrolytic stability of all candidate materials.

Hydrolysis can be defined as a double decomposition reaction that depends upon the presence of ions formed from water [1]. Since water ionizes to a greater degree as the system deviates from neutral pH, hydrolysis can be expected to proceed more rapidly under acidic or alkaline conditions. Therefore, two reasons can be postulated for the hydrolytic instability of polyester-based polymers: first, the carbon-oxygen double bond is highly polar in nature; and, second, because polyesters are, of necessity, manufactured under acidic conditions, they tend to retain some unreacted acids. This residual amount of acid further catalyzes the mechanism of hydrolytic degradation. The result is a chemical chain reaction that autocatalyzes chain scission within the polymer network.

Hydrolytic attack and degradation obey Arrhenius' Law; i.e., the rate of degradation doubles for each 10°C increase in temperature. The hydrolytic stability of the candidate materials is evaluated in accelerated fashion by subjecting the samples to 80°C isotonic saline. With chemical reaction rates doubling for each 10°C increase over body temperature, the acceleration would be $2^4 = 16$. If the samples are allowed to remain under continuous immersion for a maximum of 1100 hr, the equivalent time at physiologic temperature is 733 days, or approximately 2 years.

Based on this postulation, we can monitor any possible reduction in physical properties by plotting the percent retention of tensile strength against hours in the incubator, as shown in Figure 2. Illustrated in the graph are two hypothetical materials, A and B. Sample A can be seen to retain physical properties after 1200 hr of exposure. By contrast, Sample B has lost a significant amount of strength at the end of these tests, and would therefore be suspected of hydrolytic susceptibility. Sample B will be rejected. Sample A will be allowed to proceed to more complex tests.

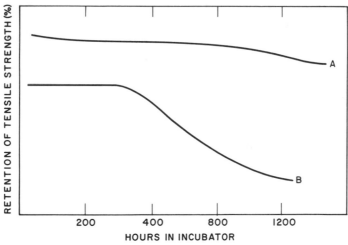

Figure 2. Accelerated hydrolytic stability test.

Oxidative Stability

Low molecular weight organic moieties are no less susceptible to oxidation than are organic polymers [2]. It is the exponential loss in physical properties due to reduction in polymer molecular weight that makes this phenomenon appear more vivid.

Because oxidation is a free radical reaction, it is governed by the same sequence of reactions found in free radical polymerization, i.e., initiation, propagation, termination and chain scission [3].

Initiation

1.1 Primary

$$PH \quad \frac{\text{Heat and/or}}{\text{UV Light Energy}} \quad P\cdot + \cdot H$$

$$PH + O_2 \qquad\qquad\qquad P\cdot + \cdot OOH$$

1.2 Secondary

A) $POOH \rightarrow PO\cdot + \cdot OH$
B) Metal-induced peroxide decomposition

$$POOH + M^{++} \rightarrow PO\cdot + M^{+++} + OH^-$$
$$POOH + M^{+++} \rightarrow POO\cdot + M^{++} + H^+$$

PH = Polymer molecule   M = Metal ion

Propagation

2.1 $\quad P\cdot + O^2 \rightarrow POO\cdot$
$\qquad POO\cdot + PH \rightarrow POOH + P\cdot$

2.2 Chain branching (autocatalytic)

$$PO\cdot + PH \rightarrow POH + P\cdot$$
$$HO\cdot + PH \rightarrow H_2O + P\cdot$$

Termination and/or Crosslinking

$P \cdot + P \cdot)$
$PO \cdot + P \cdot)$
$POO \cdot + P \cdot)$ Radical free products
$POO \cdot + PO \cdot)$
$POO \cdot + POO \cdot)$

Chain Scission

4.1 By radical decomposition

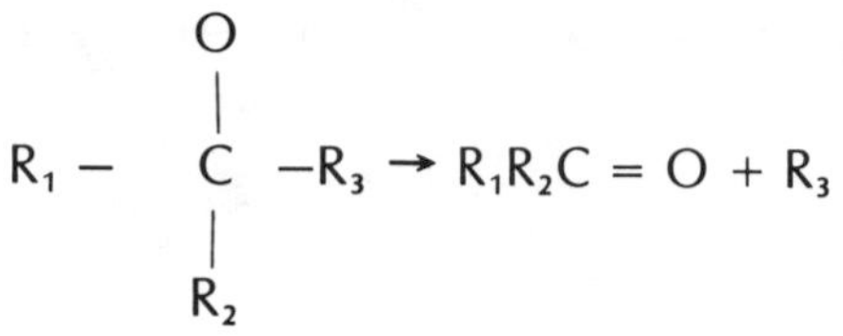

$$R_1 - \overset{\overset{\displaystyle O}{|}}{\underset{\underset{\displaystyle R_2}{|}}{C}} - R_3 \rightarrow R_1R_2C = O + R_3$$

4.2 By photolysis

$$-CH_2-CH_2-CH_2-\overset{\overset{\displaystyle O}{||}}{C}-CH_2-CH_2 + h\nu$$

$$-CH_2-CH_2-\overset{\overset{\displaystyle O}{||}}{C}\cdot + \cdot CH_2CH_2-$$

$$-CH = CH_2 + CH_3-\overset{\overset{\displaystyle O}{||}}{C}-CH_2-CH_2$$

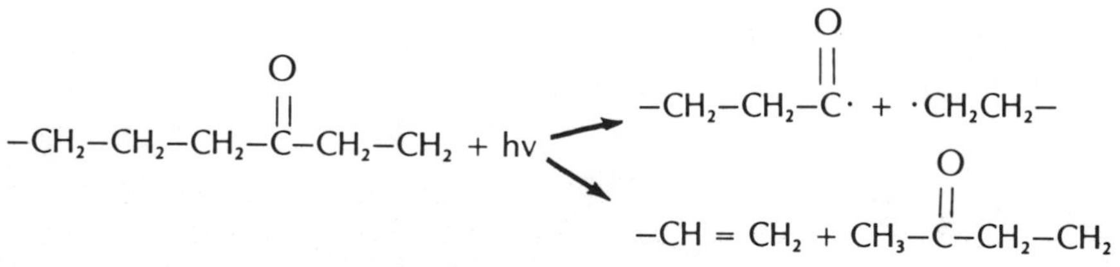

Our accelerated test for oxidative stability involves the use of an oxygen bomb apparatus. Specimens are preconditioned at 23°C, 72-percent RH in a dessicator for one week before starting the test. Specimens are exposed to an oxygen pressure of 300 psi for 30 days at

70°C; physical properties of the exposed samples are then compared to an unexposed control. Parameters measured are tensile strength, elongation at break, and tear resistance.

These test conditions were selected, since natural rubber becomes crumbly in 21 days [4]. Polyurethanes are less susceptible to oxidation than is natural rubber, but are still degraded to some extent. Therefore, we reject candidate polymers that show a decrease of 25 percent or more in tensile properties.

Another method useful in examining the oxidative degradation cascade is to compare absorbance spectra from an infrared spectrophotometer. By monitoring the intensity of the carbonyl absorption at 1709 cm^{-1}, and the methylene absorption at 1449 cm^{-1}, the ratio of the two absorptions can be used to estimate the relative extent of reaction [5].

Infrared (IR) Spectroscopy

IR spectroscopy is a powerful analytical technique used to identify chemical groups. It does so by measuring the rotational and vibrational energy of molecules. Certain functional groups exhibit "group frequency" oscillations when subjected to the energizing effect of light of specific wavenumber. These vibrational spectra can then be used as "fingerprints" to identify molecular species or to model polymer systems.

Our analytical uses of IR spectroscopy can be described as identification of fundamental chemical bonds, quantitative analysis, and a criterion for purity. We use IR spectroscopy to characterize polymers in the virgin state; following exposure to biological media, the material is rescanned for signs of possible degradation.

Attenuated Total Reflectance (ATR)

IR spectroscopy, described above, depends on the ability of a polymer to be solvated in some solvent system. The solution containing the polymer/solvent blend can then be made ready for the instrument. However, not all polymers are solvent-soluble. Many plastics are merely swollen in the presence of solvents; others, such as cross-linked polymers, are simply insoluble in common organic solvents. Whenever insoluble polymers are encountered, ATR (a variation of the IR technique) is frequently utilized.

ATR is based on the principle that, when a light beam is reflected at the interface between two parallel materials of differing refractive indexes, an evanescent wave is obtained, propagating across the surfaces. The propagating wave is slightly absorbed by the specimen, producing an attenuated reflection. When the number of reflections are increased and plotted as a function of wavelength by the instrument, an absorption spectrum characteristic of the material surface is obtained [6,7]. This principle is depicted in Figure 3.

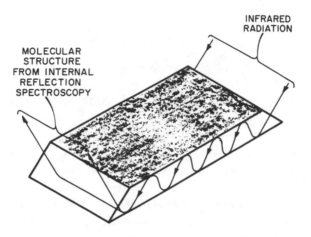

INFRARED
RADIATION

MOLECULAR
STRUCTURE
FROM INTERNAL
REFLECTION
SPECTROSCOPY

Figure 3. Attenuated total reflectance.

We obtain attenuated surface spectra of candidate biomaterials, before and after biological exposure, by means of a Wilks Model 10 ATR accessory. After biological exposure, particular attention is paid to any degradative signs on the material surface. These observations are considered to be exceptionally significant since many degradative effects are initially concentrated on the surface. Recognition of preliminary surface effects may lead to predictions of long-term material stability in a physiological environment. ATR is particularly useful for the detection and identification of surface contaminants such as mold release agents, surface oxidation, and degradation due to thermal processing.

Gel Permeation Chromatography (GPC)

A common effect realized from all modes of polymer degradation is a decrease in the number average and perhaps the weight average molecular weight. Attention is frequently called to the generalized rela-

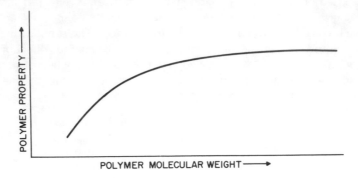

Figure 4. General relationship of polymer properties and molecular weight.

tionship of polymer molecular weight and properties, as shown in Figure 4.

Generally, a decrease in molecular weight is followed by a drastic deterioration in physical properties. Thus, a means of recording degradation could be crudely derived from stress-strain data. However, the rate and extent of deterioration could be relatively small, and the response could be masked by normal experimental scatter. Fortunately, a more accurate and acceptable method of quantitatively assaying minor shifts in both weight and number average molecular weights can be found in GPC.

GPC separates molecules according to size. The method has therefore found wide application in the study of molecular weight distributions. Polymers are heterogeneous in molecular weight; i.e., they contain a wide range of molecular weights from which certain averages can be calculated. Polymers are generally characterized by the number average ($\overline{M}_n$) and weight average ($\overline{M}_w$). Molecular weights were

$$M_n = \frac{\sum\limits_{i=1}^{\infty} N_i M_i}{\sum\limits_{i=1}^{\infty} N_i}$$

and

$$\overline{M}_w = \frac{\displaystyle\sum_{i=1}^{\infty} N_i \overline{M}^2{}_i}{\displaystyle\sum_{i=1}^{\infty} N_i \overline{M}_i}$$

The ratio of $\overline{M}_w/\overline{M}_n$ measures the polydispersity of the material and can vary in value from 1.5 to 50. The closer the ratio is to 1.5, the narrower the molecular weight distribution of a given polymer. This is usually considered a desirable characteristic in polymers, and in biomaterials in particular, since low molecular weight fractions could migrate from the polymer to the surrounding blood stream [8]. Determination of molecular weight and distribution is crucial in polymer work.

In principle, GPC determines molecular weight by separating molecules on the basis of size alone. A polymer solution is forced to pass through a packed column of controlled pore size. The larger molecules (higher molecular weight) will elute first, and the smaller molecules (lower molecular weight) will elute last. If the eluting stream is connected to an appropriate detector and chart recorder, a series of peaks will result. Times and peak heights are characteristic of molecular weight and concentration, respectively. A typical chromatogram is shown in Figure 5. Peak 1 is a bell-shaped curve, corresponding to a Gaussian distribution of the various molecular weights that comprise the polymer. Curves 2 and 3 represent low molecular weight additives.

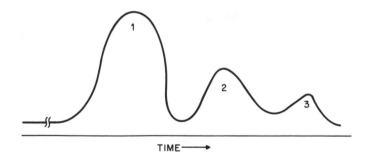

TIME→

Figure 5. A typical chromatogram.

$\overline{M}_w$ and $\overline{M}_n$ can be closely approximated by comparing obtained values to a standard curve constructed from model polystyrene samples of known molecular weight. Polystyrene is generally used because the mechanics of polymerization allow samples of narrow molecular weight distribution to be obtained. Styrene reference samples of varying molecular weights are run through the columns, giving a characteristic elution volume. A plot relating volume versus molecular weight can then be constructed, as shown in Figure 6.

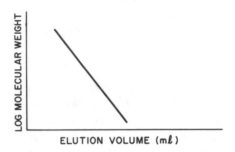

Figure 6. *Elution volume versus molecular weight for styrene.*

From this plot, the approximate molecular weight of an unknown sample can be estimated by determining its elution volume, and reading the molecular weight from the calibration curve. It should be noted that the molecular weights obtained by this method are only approximate, since the calibration curves were obtained empirically from styrene polymer. The actual values of $\overline{M}_n$ and $\overline{M}_w$ can be determined through intrinsic viscosity measurements.

Intrinsic viscosity measurements are derived from rheological data (see section of Physical Chemical Characterization). Intrinsic viscosity is related to viscosity average molecular weight by the expression

$$[\eta] = K^1 M_v^a$$

As a approaches unity, viscosity average molecular weight ($\overline{M}_v$) is approximately equal to weight average molecular weight ($\overline{M}_w$) [9].

Thus, from intrinsic viscosity, the absolute weight average molecular weight can be calculated for any polymer. This information can then be used in GPC to measure $\overline{M}_w$ from instrument response.

GPC is an invaluable tool for determining polymer properties. Its technique for separations based upon molecular sizes is well established.

For applications involving separation of components or a simple comparison of samples, measurement of the retention volume is all that is necessary. However, if molecular weight determinations are desired, calibration by any of the following methods can be done: "Q-Factor", "Benoit", or "Unperturbed dimensions". Dawkins has done a fine review on all three methods [10].

Differential Scanning Calorimetry

Differential thermal analysis (DTA) and differential scanning calorimetry (DSC) are techniques that measure enthalpy changes of a polymer as a function of temperature. DSC is considered a quantitative version of DTA and the terms are often used interchangeably. Typical applications include determination of percent crystallinity, degree of polymer blends and copolymers, and measurements of transition temperatures such as melting point and glass transition temperature [11].

Figure 7 is an operation schematic of a DSC instrument [12]. It explains how enthalpy change in the sample being energized is measured in comparison to the reference temperature. The measure of heat flow versus sample temperature is also shown in Figure 7. This is a small portion of a typical curve obtained by DSC analysis; a complete curve showing the resolution of melting points, T_g, and extent of crystallinity is depicted in Figure 8.

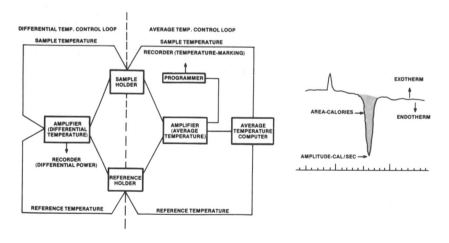

Figure 7. Block diagram of a differential scanning calorimeter and a typical chart record.

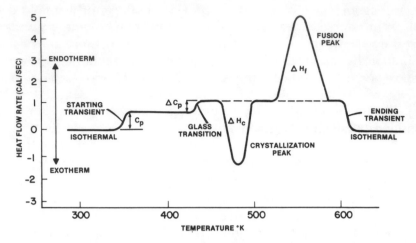

Figure 8. Schematic representation of DSC output (reproduced from Operators Manual, DSC-2, Perkin Elmer Corp., Norwalk, Conn.)

Two problems using the DSC instrument lie in the areas of 1) establishment of an accurate base line necessary for quantitative measurement, and 2) accurate initial weighing of the sample. If the sample is weighed out to four decimal places, an accuracy of reproducibility ± percent can be obtained [13]. A method for determining the base line is described by Bascom [14].

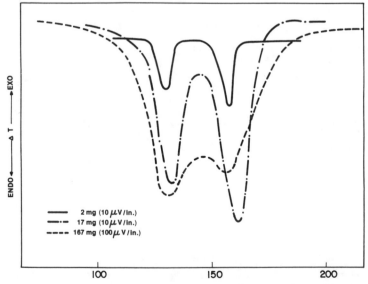

Figure 9. DTA of 25:75 Polyethylene:Propylene blend; heating rate, 45°C/min [15].

Our primary reasons for using the DSC analysis method are: data determined by other types of analysis can be correlated; insoluble specimens may be used; no special shape of the specimen is necessary; and sample size can be very small. In fact, Figure 9 shows that smaller sample weights yield higher resolution of DTA data [15].

The DSC technique for characterizing polymers is well documented [16]. This method can be used to determine the purity of a sample, the transition points, and, when needed, the extents of reactions. DSC has the sensitivity to accurately measure subtle property changes or effects not readily discernible by other forms of analysis.

PHYSICAL CHEMICAL ANALYSES

Polymer solutions show a marked increase in viscosity when compared with the pure solvent. This increase is apparent even at concentrations as low as 0.5 percent [17]. This positive change in viscosity is attributable to several parameters, one of which is the molecular weight of the polymer. This dependence is the basis for molecular weight determinations by solution rheology and intrinsic viscosity techniques.

Viscosity is a measure of the solution rheology of a particular system. Rheology is the science of the deformation and flow of matter. It describes the behavior of substances that flow when subjected to shear stress. The basic relationship, $v = \eta D$, mathematically defines the shear stress, v, with the shear rate, D.

The equation $v = \eta D$ is known as Newton's Law. This relationship assumes a linear correlation between v and D, with η being a constant. If liquids behave in this fashion, they are known as Newtonian liquids; but this is only an idealized concept. In reality, few liquids behave in this fashion. More than 90 percent of all liquids are non-Newtonian [18]. The flow behavior of liquids can be described by the curves in Figure 10.

Intrinsic viscosity is an algebraic manipulation derived from rheological data. The well-known Mark-Houwink expression [19] relates intrinsic viscosity, η, to weight average molecular weight, $\overline{M}_w$. The relationship is expressed as

$$[\eta] = K^1 M_w^a$$

where K^1 and a are constants determined from a plot of $\ln[\eta]$ versus $\ln \overline{M}_n$. K^1 is the ordinate intercept and a is the slope of the curve. This graph is shown in Figure 11.

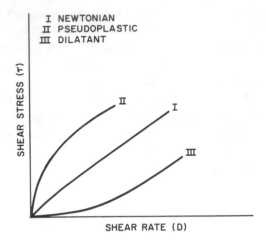

Figure 10. Flow behavior of liquids.

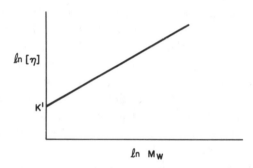

Figure 11. Graphic representation of Mark-Houwink expression [18].

The experimental procedure consists of: 1) measuring the efflux time (v) required for a given volume of polymer solution to flow through a capillary viscometer (Figure 12) and 2) relating it to the corresponding efflux time (v_o) for the solvent. This leads to the following expressions:

Relative Viscosity $\eta_r = \eta/\eta_o = v/v_o$
Specific Viscosity $\eta_{sp} = \eta_{rel} - 1$
Reduced Viscosity $\eta_{red} = \eta_{sp}/C$
Inherent Viscosity $\eta_{inh} = 1n\ \eta_{rel}/C$
Intrinsic Viscosity $[\eta] = (\eta_{sp}/C)C = 0$

The last expression is graphically shown in Figure 13. Once intrinsic

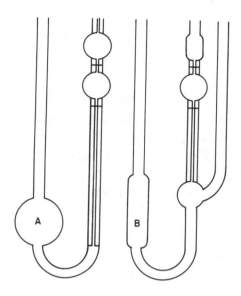

Figure 12. The Ostwald (a) and Ubbelohde suspended level (b) viscometers.

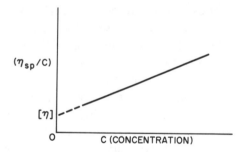

Figure 13. Determination of intrinsic viscosity.

viscosity has been determined for a given polymer/solvent pair, it can be used to calculate molecular weights of unknown polymers.

The determination of polymer molecular weight can be carried out quickly and accurately by making use of a capillary viscometer. Polymers in very dilute solutions behave as Newtonian fluids; thus, their viscosities can readily be determined by capillary methods. The cost of this comparatively simple apparatus is negligible when compared to more sophisticated forms of testing. It is this simplicity and lower cost that makes this procedure attractive in polymer analytical procedures.

Our molecular weight determinations are used to provide a datum line for all polymers intended as medical implants; following explanation, possible degradations can be detected by downward shifts in molecular weight distributions.

MECHANICAL PROPERTIES

There are a number of analytical techniques for evaluating the mechanical properties of polymers. Two of the most useful are stress-strain analysis, and dynamic mechanical analysis. The former is an established American Society for Testing of Materials (ASTM) procedure that has been modified for polymer characterization; the latter is a relatively new method of characterizing polymers by mechanical properties.

Stress-Strain Analysis

The stress-strain test is perhaps the most widely used of all mechanical tests. This is usually done by measuring continuously the force developed as the sample is elongated at a constant rate of extension. Stress-strain tests give an indication not only of the strength of a material, but also of its toughness. The concept of toughness may be defined in several ways, one of which is in terms of the area under the stress-strain curve. Toughness, therefore, is an indication of the energy that a material is capable of absorbing before breaking. Thus, the larger the area under the curve, the "tougher" the material.

The generalized stress-strain curve shown in Figure 14 serves to define several useful quantities such as modulus of elasticity, yield stress, and elongation at break [20]. The slope of the initial straight-line portion of the curve is the modulus of elasticity. In a tensile test, this modulus is Young's Modulus. Mathematically, it is defined as

$$E = \frac{d\sigma}{d\varepsilon}$$

The maximum in the curve denotes the stress yield, σy, and the elongation at yield, εy. The end of the curve denotes the failure of the material, which is characterized by tensile strength, σB, and the ultimate strain or elongation at break, ε_B. If Hooke's Law holds, the elastic modulus is defined by:

$$\tau = E\varepsilon$$

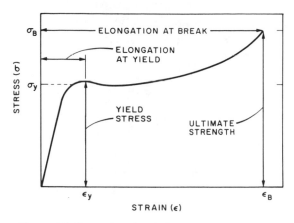

Figure 14. Generalized Tensile Stress-Strain Curve.

and each of increasing technical complexity. If a material fails to meet required specifications at critical points, provisions are made for immediate acceptance/rejection decisions.

Candidate polymers are first characterized in their virgin state to establish a datum reference line. Following this primary series of tests, the material is subjected to in vitro and in vivo degradation tests; the exposed specimens are then re-examined for possible mechanical or chemical degradation. Underlying this protocol is the assumption that testing candidate materials in the virgin state, and retesting after exposure to challenging biological environments, will reveal both desirable and undesirable properties.

Figure 1 defines the Evaluation Protocol. The initial stages of the screening process are accomplished by a combination of carefully selected validity trials. Recommendation points are provided after finalizing preliminary screening tests; these decision points are designed to preclude an unfit material from proceeding into biological exposure tests. The biological test matrix is performed only after a candidate biomaterial has successfully passed all previous requirements. The test matrix followed at Thermo Electron is summarized in Table 1.

It should be pointed out that the test battery focuses on both static and dynamic material properties. Initial tests are accelerated, progressing to long-term, actual-configuration bladder endurance runs or heated circulatory analog loops.

This approach provides two important advantages: First, analysis of the generated data provides meaningful comparisons among competing biomaterials. Second, this test format can form the basis for a Quality Control Program. After a biomaterial has been accepted, the principal objective of this type of testing is the reproducibility of results from one manufacturing lot to the next.

Where

$$\sigma = \frac{\text{force or load F}}{\text{cross-sectional area A}}$$

$$\varepsilon = \frac{\text{L-Lo}}{\text{Lo}} \quad \frac{\Delta L}{\text{Lo}}$$

All our stress-strain data are obtained in an Istron Extensometer by following a modified ASTM D412-66 procedure which provides a convenient set of data useful in quality control and as an indication of polymer degradation following implantation.

Dynamic Mechanical Analysis

Dynamic mechanical testing yields more intrinsic information about a polymer than any other single measurement. Dynamic mechanical analysis, along with microscopic and other spectroscopic techniques, represents one of the most comprehensive analytical techniques for polymer characterization [21].

The term "dynamic property" generally applies to the linear viscoelastic response of a polymer to an externally applied frequency; when the frequency and temperature are varied, a spectrum of responses can be obtained. The Rheovibron is an instrument designed to measure the time dependence of viscoelastic materials [22]. To accomplish this end, it imposes a small oscillatory sine wave (or strain) or low amplitude so that the response of the sample is within linear range.

The tests usually consist of placing a thin film of test material with the temperature adjusted to any desired value. The sample is next subjected to a small sinusoidal strain wave with the response measured in terms of load on the phase angle between the sinusoidal strain input and the sinusoidal stress output.

The phase angle, which reflects the time lag between the applied stress and strain, is δ, and it is defined by a ratio called the dissipation factor [23]:

$$\tan \delta = G''/G'$$

where G' is a real modulus, and G'' is an imaginary modulus. The real and imaginary moduli are defined by a complex modulus of the following form:

$$G^* = G' + iG''$$

where G^* is the complex shear modulus, and $i = \sqrt{-1}$.

The size of the phase angle (tan δ) is a direct measure of how elastic or how viscous the test material is. If the phase angle is $0°$, the material is perfectly elastic (ideal spring). If the material is completely viscous, the phase angle is $90°$. In other words, in elastic systems, all the work is stored as potential energy, as in a stretched spring; by distinction, in a totally viscous system, all the work done on the system is dissipated as heat. Most elastomers fall somewhere between these two extremes. Ideally, a bladder material should have as small an angle as possible (purely elastic) to be capable of withstanding prolonged and continuous flexing.

The Rheovibron automatically computes tan δ and conveniently displays the value as a gauge readout. Tan δ at physiologic temperatures as a significant data point useful for understanding the viscoelastic flow of a polymer. The Rheovibron instrument is shown in Figure 15.

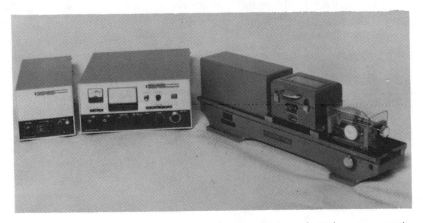

Figure 15. Rheovibron Viscoelastometer. Photograph shows base frame supporting the electromechanical driver unit, stress-strain transducer and temperature control chamber; a console containing the amplifier and oscillator chassis, the tan δ meter, and the main controls; and the power supply to the instrument.

The Rheovibron can also be used to determine the nature of a given copolymer or blend. The dynamic response of a random copolymer will generally fall between those of the individual homopolymers. The presence of significant blocks of either component will appear as damping maxima at temperatures corresponding to the individual transitions of the respective homopolymers. A broad damping peak and a gradual modulus drop with temperature are characteristics of heterogeneous copolymerization, whereas a narrow damping peak with a sharp drop in modulus would indicate a homogeneous copolymerization.

By the same token, the dynamic mechanical behavior of polymer blends is quite analogous to that described for copolymers. Incompatible or multiphase clends tend to show the characteristics of all components present and are, to a limited degree, consistent with the concentration of a particular component.

The Rheovibron can also be used to study the chemical compatibility of homopolymers, copolymers, and blends. If the constituents are mutually soluble, the transitions should amalgamate. If the components are mutually insoluble, two transition points can be expected.

The Rheovibron is basically a dynamic spectrometer that "massages" the molecules of the material at low amplitudes of strain, and measures their response. Usually, instruments are run purely on a temperature scan, since most investigators are simply interested in determining where T_g and T_m occur at a fixed frequency.

The Rheovibron is designed to scan temperatures from $-100\,°C$ to $+200\,°C$, monitor the change in the phase angle, and measure modulus. For most typical elastomers, whenever a major transition point is reached, the modulus can change by as much as three decades in magnitude [24]. Under these conditions, the modulus decreases drastically while, at the same time, the dissipation of energy in the sample or loss angle, δ, goes through a maximum [25]. In this fashion, transition temperatures can be detected, measured, and defined.

Mechanical testing of polymers by the stress-strain method and the dynamic mechanical analysis is generally faster and lends a clearer indication of polymer performance, as compared to other forms of mechanical testing.

Mock Loop Testing

Fatigue can be defined as many material failure or degradation of mechanical properties due to oscillatory deformations or stresses [26]. There are many types of fatigue testers, ranging from tensile or flexural tests, to rotating beam instruments [27].

As elastomers replace metals and other materials in critical applications, fatigue tests become increasingly important since the maximum oscillatory load that elastomers are capable of sustaining is only a fraction of its tensile strength [28]. Thus, the more conventional tests give little indication of the lifetime of a material subjected to vibrations or repeated deformations.

Long-term in vitro testing is essential in the development and testing of a reliable cardiac assist device. In our laboratories [29], we have carefully evaluated those requirements deemed necessary to properly design a real-time testing facility. The most important characteristics that must be controlled and monitored are as follows:

- Viscosity of the fluid
- Flow rate of the fluid
- Pump fill pressure
- Pump outlet pressure
- Fluid temperature
- Fluid salinity
- Pump beat rate
- Pump systole/diastole ratio
- Mechanical compliance system to reflect the animal compliance system
- Flexibility of individual pump testing

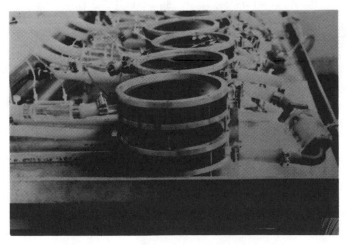

Figure 16. Close-up view of test substation.

Thermo Electron maintains a testing facility capable of evaluating 64 pumps simultaneously, designed and built to reflect the above requirements. Figure 16 illustrates one of several identical test substations currently in operation, with each substation capable of testing 16 individual pumps. Each substation contains its own independent fluid manifold assembly with its own fluid temperature regulator.

Figure 17 is a partial view of the testing facility, showing the compliance bags, transparent pump housings, and ancillary control equipment. Figure 18 shows typical geometries of axisymmetric blood pumps used clinically and experimentally.

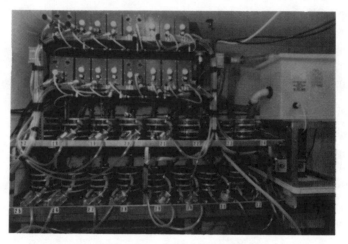

Figure 17. Partial view of mock loop test facility.

HEMOCOMPATIBILITY

The successful development of blood pumps suitable for use in cardiac assist devices is a long and involved process, a most important aspect of which is the hemocompatibility of the polymer intended for use as the bladder. Kusserow, et al. [30] state that the safety of any prosthetic device is open to serious question until it has been conclusively demonstrated that its blood-contacting surfaces do not cause embolic episodes.

Investigators agree that adsorption of plasma proteins is the first in a complex series of events that occur when a synthetic material is placed in

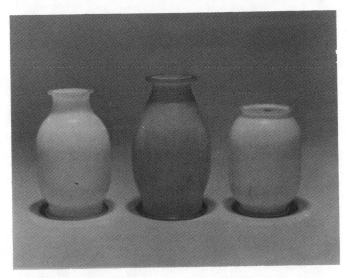

Figure 18. Axisymmetric blood pumps used clinically and experimentally.

the cardiovascular system [31-33]. Bruck [34] concludes that this process seems to be completed in less than 3 sec, and that it effectively influences the subsequent interactions of the formed blood elements, especially platelets with the proteinated surfaces. Vroman, et al. [35] reported that adsorbed proteins can be enzymatically degraded and replaced by other proteins, or they can undergo various conformational and configurated changes, in addition to destruction. These changes induce platelet aggregation and activation of the blood coagulation cascade, resulting in thrombus formation. If thrombus particles are dislodged from the surface, life-threatening emboli can occur.

Investigations conducted at the Department of Pathology of the University of Vermont suggesting the following:

Implantation of synthetic surfaces into the vascular system may bring about the formation of emboli in both direct and indirect fashion. The direct mechanism of prosthesis-induced embolism induces the initial formation of a thromboembolic deposit on the surface of the implant, followed by loosening and dislodgement of embolic particles into the blood stream. The indirect mechanism is thought to involve the formation of minute platelet and fibrin emboli within the blood stream itself, due possibly to the release of thromboplastin corpuscles. This process is analogous to that seen in certain instances of disseminated intravascular coagulation. There may be resultant microinfarction of the tissues and varying depletion of primary clotting factors. It is evident that an important relation may exist between prosthesis-induced thromboembolic phenomena and blood trauma [36].

Table 2. Selected Hemocompatibility Tests.

Modality	Technique	Monitored Parameter(s)
In vitro	Ellipsometry [37-39]	Fibrinogen, serum albumin, γ-globulin
In vitro and Ex vivo	Rotating Disc [40,41]	Shear-induced hemolysis, platelet adhesion, radioautographic visualization of adsorbed labelled proteins.
Ex vivo	Couette-type [42] test chamber	Formation rate and composition of thrombus.
In vitro	Kinetic blood [43] coagulation test	Weight of formed thrombus amount of unclotted, platelet reduction.
Ex vivo	Stagnation point [44-46] Flow Experiment	Blood interfacial effects.
In vivo	Vena Cava [47] Ring Test	Presence of thrombi
In vivo	Renal Embolus [48] Test	Renal bed utilized as indicator for thromboembolic events originating at test ring.

The determination of blood compatibility is thus a multifaceted task; no single measurement provides an unequivocal answer. Therefore, we feel hemocompatibility should be ascertained by a battery of tests. Table 2 summarizes some current techniques. It should be emphasized, however, that the list is not meant to be all-inclusive; rather, it is designed to provide a reasonable cross section of accepted methodology. Furthermore, test procedures are covered only superficially; the reader is directed to the original source for an in-depth explanation of responses.

REFERENCES

1. Bolger, J.C., Treatise on Adhesion and Adhesives, Vol. 3, Marcel Dekker, New York, p. 8 (1973).
2. Dubin, P.L., J. Soc. Plst. Eng., 10:29 (1977).
3. Abramoff, C.S., Modern Plastics Encyclopedia, Vol. 54, No. 10A, McGraw-Hill, New York, p. 144 (1978).

4. Remington, W.J. and Walsh, R.H., *Urethane Resilient Foam From Polyesters*, E.I. Du-Pont Bul. HR-10 (1956).

5. Wilkes Scientific Corp., *Recommended Practices for Internal Reflection Spectroscopy*, 1965.

6. Harrick, N.S., *Internal Reflection Spectroscopy*, John Wiley & Sons, New York (1967).

7. Wilkes Scientific Corp., *Internal Reflection Spectroscopy*, Vol. 1 (1965).

8. Kim, S.W., *Applied Chemistry at Protein Interfaces*, ACS Pub. No. 145, Chap. 10 (1975).

9. Billmeyer, F.W., *Polymer Science*, Interscience Publishers, New York, p. 83 (1962).

10. Dawkins, J.V., "Calibration Procedures in Gel Permeation Chromatography," Br. Polymer J., 4:87-101 (1972).

11. Bremman, W.P., MPL, 98 (1979).

12. Watson, E.S., O'Neill, M.J., Justin, J., and Brenner, N., Amal. Chem., 36,:1233 (1964).

13. Slade, S.E. and Jenkins, L.T., *Thermal Characterization Techniques*, Marcel Dekker, New York, p. 13 (1970).

14. Bascom, W.D. and Peyser, P., *Polymer Characterization Using Differential Scanning Techniques*, Naval Research Laboratory.

15. Chiu, J., *Polymer Characterization by Thermal Methods of Analysis*, Marcel Dekker, New York, p. 7 (1974).

16. Frazer, A.H., *High Temperature Resistent Polymers*, Wiley Intersciences, New York, 1968.

17. Margerison, B., *Introduction to Polymer Chemistry*, Pergamon Press, New York, p. 101 (1967).

18. Schramm, G., *An Introduction to Rheology and Viscometry*, Haake Tech. Bull.

19. Ravve, A., *Organic Chemistry of Macromolecules*, Marcel Dekker, New York, 1967.

20. Billmeyer, F.W., *Testbook of Polymer Science*, Interscience Publishers, New York, 1966.

21. Kuo, G.P., *Plastics Engineering*, Vol. 30, No. 5 (1974).

22. Takayanagi, M., *Proceedings Fourth International Congress on Rheology*, 1965.

23. Nielsen, L.E., *Mechanical Properties of Polymers and Composites*, Vol. 1, Marcel Dekker, New York, 1974.

24. Smith, T.L., *Molecular and Phenomenological Aspects of Rubber Elasticity and Viscoelasticity*, presented at meeting of Society of Rheology, New York, 1977.

25. Kajiyama, T., *ACS Polymer Preprints*, Vol. 10, No. 1 (1969).

26. Dillon, J.H., *Advances in Colloid Sciences*, Vol. 3, Chap. 3, Mark, H. and Verney, E.J., Eds., Interscience Pub. Inc., New York, p. 219 (1950).

27. Lazam, B.J. and Yorgiadis, A., Symposium on Plastics Spec. Tech. Pub. No. 59, Phil., Am. Soc. Testing Materials, p. 66 (February 1944).

28. Nielsen, L.E., *Mechanical Properties of Polymers*, Chapter 9, Reinhold Pub. Corp., New York, p. 231 (1967).

29. Keiser, J.T. and Bernhard, W.F., *Development and Evaluation of Unilateral and Bilateral Cardiac Assist Devices*, Annual Report NO-HT-4-2910, NTIS, Aug. 1974.

30. Kusserow, B.K. and Larrow, R.W., *Analysis and Measurements of the Effects of Materials on Blood Leukocytes, Erythrocytes, and Platelets*, Annual Report No. NO1-HB-5929-5, NTIS, January 1976.

31. Vroman, L. and Adams, A.L., J. Biomed. Mater. Res., 3:43 (1969).

32. Dutton, R.C., Weber, A.J., Johnson, A.S., and Baier, R.E., J. Biomed. Mater. Res., *3*:13 (1969).
33. Lyman, D.J., Brash, J.L., Chaikin, S.W., Klein, K.G., and Carini, M., Trans. ASAIO, *14*:250 (1968).
34. Bruck, S.D., J. Biomed. Mater. Res. Symposium, *8*:2 (1977).
35. Vroman, K., Adams, A.L., and Klings, M., Proc. Fed. Amer. Soc. Exp. Biol., *30*:1494 (1971).
36. Kusserow, B.K. and Larrow, R.W., *Analysis and Measurements of the Effects of Materials on Blood Leukocytes, Erythrocytes, and Platelets,* Annual Report No. NO1-HB-5929-5, NTIS, January 1976.
37. McCrackin, F.L., Passaglia, E., Stromberg, R.R., and Steinberg, H.L., J. Res. Natl. Bur. Std., *A67*:363 (1963).
38. Fenstermaker, C.A., Grant, W.H., Morrissey, B.W., Smith, L.E., and Stromberg, R.R., *Interaction of Plasma Proteins with Surfaces,* Annual Report No. PB 232-629, NTIS, March 1974.
39. Morrissey, B.W., Smith, L.E., Fenstermaker, C.A., Stromberg, R.R., and Grant, W.H., "Confirmation of Adsorbed Blood Proteins" Proc. Symp. of AAMI, NBS Spec. Publ. 415, New Orleans, 1974.
40. Williams, M.C., *The Influence of Biomaterials and Blood Chemistry on Shear-Induced Hemolysis,* University of California, Annual Report No. NIH-NO1-HV-3-2952-4 NTIS, August 1976.
41. Leonard, E.F., Kochwa, S., Lauren, M.D., Litwak, R.S., and Rosenfield, R.E., *Coordinated Studies of Platelet and Protein Reactions on Artificial Materials,* Columbia University, Annual Report No. NO1-HV-3-2910-3, NTIS, August 1976.
42. Schultz, J.S., Ciarkowski, A.A., Goddard, I.D., Penner, J.S., and Lindenauer, S.M., *Evaluation of the Compatibility of Materials in Contact with Blood,* University of Michigan, Annual Report No. NO1-HB-4-2962-2, NTIS, July 1976.
43. Kambic, H.E., Kiraly, R.J., and Nose, Y., J. Biomed. Mater. Res. Sump., *7*:561-570 (1976).
44. Petscheck, H.E., Adamis, D., and Kantrowitz, A.R., Trans. ASAIO, *14*:256 (1968).
45. Madras, P.N., Morton, W.A., and Petschek, H.E., FEd. Proc., *30*:1665 (1971).
46. Morton, W.A., Nyilas, E., Herzlinger, G.A., and Petschek, H.E., Circulation, *50* (Suppl III):297 (1974).
47. Daniels, A.J., Mortensen, I.O., and Grahn, A.R., *Vena Cava Ring Tests of Biomaterials in Dogs,* Utah Biomedical Test Laboratory, Annual Report No. NO1-HV-6-2911-1, NTIS, August 1976.
48. Harris, L.S., Craighead, J.E., and Larrow, R., *Evaluation of Materials for Their Thromboembolic and Blood Trauma Effects,* University of Vermont, Annual Report No. NO1-HV-5-2939-6, NTIS, August 1976.

SYNTHESIS AND BIOMEDICAL APPLICATIONS
OF POLYURETHANES

Henri Ulrich, Henry W. Bonk and George C. Colovos

The Upjohn Company
Donald S. Gilmore Research Laboratories
North Haven, Connecticut 06473

INTRODUCTION

Polyurethanes are a unique class of polymers because an infinite variety of products with a wide range of physical properties are readily synthesized from liquid components at room temperature. The basic reaction consists of polyaddition of a di or polyisocyanate to a polyester or polyether based di or polyol to give products ranging from soft elastomers to rigid foams. Presently approximately 35 million pounds of polyurethane per year are being used for medical devices and rapid growth is expected, especially when researchers and manufacturers become more sophisticated in tailoring the basic polyurethane products to the intended application.

Polyurethane elastomers, for example, are important materials for artificial heart and kidney components, surgical prostheses, catheters, and artificial blood vessels, and they are beginning to replace silicone, polyvinyl chloride and methyl methacrylate to restore facial features. Polyurethane elastomers have also been successfully applied in heart assist devices, in the fabrication of tubing for hemodialysis units and for intravenous feeding kits, and in the construction of blood bags and solution containers. Recent data indicate that they may also become quite useful in the formulation of hemostatic coatings and biomedical adhesives. Flexible polyurethane foams have been proposed for the construction of bandaging materials, surgical dressings and absorbent

29

materials in general. Even rigid polyurethane foams have been utilized for casts and for prosthetic applications.

Polyurethane Elastomers

Polyurethane elastomers are either thermoplastic or thermoset materials. The latter are used as liquid cast systems, while thermoplastic polyurethane elastomers are supplied in form of solid pellets or granules intended for injection molding, blow molding or extrusion applications. All of the commercial thermoplastic polyurethane elastomers are linear segmented polymers, based on a diisocyanate, a high molecular weight diprimary diol and a glycol extender. Random melt polymerization processes are being used to manufacture these elastomers. The following general structure exemplifies thermoplastic polyurethane elastomers and variations are achieved by using different polyol backbones:

$$\left[NH-\langle\bigcirc\rangle-CH_2-\langle\bigcirc\rangle-NH-\overset{\overset{O}{\|}}{C}-O-R-O-\overset{\overset{O}{\|}}{C}-NH- \right.$$

$$\left. -\langle\bigcirc\rangle-CH_2-\langle\bigcirc\rangle-NH-\overset{\overset{O}{\|}}{C}-O-R'-O-\overset{\overset{O}{\|}}{C} \right]_n$$

The high molecular weight diprimary diols (R), which constitute the soft segments of the elastomer backbone, are summarized in Table 1. The short chain diol extenders (R') are usually 1,4-butanediol, 1,6-hexanediol, diethylene glycol and the like.

Processing aids are also incorporated in TPU's to facilitate subsequent processing. The reaction of the diisocyanate with glycol chain extender and high molecular weight diol results in the formation of hard and soft segments, respectively, with the ratio of hard to soft segments in a chain regulating hardness, modulus and elongation of the elastomers. The thus produced thermoplastic elastomers have high tensile strengths (5000-7000 psi) at high elongation (350-600%) and superior toughness and abrasion resistance. Their unique balance of physical properties is achieved by strong interchain interaction leading to domain type of chain entanglements. Upon heating and melting the chains become disoriented but domain structures reform on cooling.

Table 1. Macromolecular Diol.

$$HO(CH_2)_4 \left[O(CH_2)_4 \right]_n OH$$

Poly(tetramethylene oxide) glycol

$$HO-\underset{\underset{CH_3}{|}}{CH}-CH_2 \left[O-\underset{\underset{CH_3}{|}}{CH}CH_2 \right]_n OH$$

Poly(1,2-oxypropylene) glycol

$$HOCH_2CH_2 \left[OCH_2CH_2 \right]_n OH$$

Poly(1,2-oxyethylene) glycol

$$HO(CH_2)_4 \left[O-\underset{\underset{O}{\|}}{C}-(CH_2)_5 \right]_n OH$$

Poly(caprolactone) glycol

$$HO(CH_2)_4 \left[O-\underset{\underset{O}{\|}}{C}-(CH_2)_4-\underset{\underset{O}{\|}}{C}-O(CH_2)_4 \right]_n OH$$

Poly(tetramethylene adipate) glycol

Polyurethane elastomers fall into two groups of products, polyesters or polyethers. Products based on polycaprolactone are also available. For biomedical applications polyether based materials are preferred because of their excellent hydrolytic stability and their biological inertness. In the formulation of products for biomedical applications it is also mandatory to avoid stabilizers, catalysts and processing aids which contain toxic materials. A suitable polyether based thermoplastic polyurethane was developed by Upjohn, and a series of different hardness products are marketed under the tradename Pellethane® 2363 [1].

Pellethane 2363 has passed the class VI series of tests as specified in the USP XIX. These tests are intended to screen plastic materials suitable for use in the fabrication of biomedical products. Master files have been established in the Food and Drug Sections of FDA.

Short term toxicological tests have shown that Pellethane 2363 is in compliance with existing regulation and long term studies are in progress. These tests include tissue culture on the sample and on extracts using both mammalian and human cells, rabbit implant, hemolysis, intracutaneous injection in rabbits, systemic toxicity in mice, cell growth inhibition of the aqueous extract, total and extractable heavy metals and buffering capacity. The extracting media were saline, PEG 400, and cottonseed oil. The Cumulative Toxicity Index is less than 100, demonstrating that these products are essentially non-toxic materials under the acute toxicity tests employed [2]. In addition to the chemical and physical tests conducted routinely on manufactured thermoplastic elastomers, cytotoxicity tests are performed on every manufactured lot. The metal content of Pellethane® 2363-80A is low with the exception of tin (40 ppm) because stannous octoate is used as a catalyst to promote the reaction of the diisocyanate with the polyols. Typical physical properties of Pellethane® 2363 products are listed in Table 2.

Table 2. Typical Physical Properties of 2363 Series.

Grade	80A	90A	55D
Hardness, Shore	83A	93A	55D
Specific Gravity, g/cc	1.13	1.14	1.15
Tensile Modulus, psi			
@ 50% elongation	550	1100	1800
100% elongation	850	1530	2500
300% elongation	1650	3100	4500
Tensile Strength, psi	6000	6750	6500
Elongation at break, %	550	500	430
Tear Strength, Die C, pli	475	575	650
Compressive Stress, psi			
@ 5%	220	450	540
10%	400	650	930
25%	890	1400	2000
50%	2530	5000	6160
Clash-Berg modulus, T_F, °C.	-58	-46	-21
Taber Abrasion, H-22 Wheel, mg loss	<0.02	<0.01	<0.08

Melt processing of all thermoplastic polyurethanes requires that the material be dried prior to usage for optimal results. Dehumidifying hopper dryers are recommended for large volume production while tray drying can be used for very small volumes [3].

The equipment recommended for extruding Pellethane 2363 resins includes a single stage non-vented, 24/1 LD extruder with a heavy duty, DC variable speed, high torque drive. For example, a 2-½ inch extruder should have a 40-50 hp drive. Screw design is of the metering type (6 flights feed-9 flights transition-9 flights metering) with a 2.6-3.1 compression ratio. The employment of breaker plates and screen packs is standard operating procedure with these materials. Barrel temperatures are generally cooler at the rear depending on the extrusion product: film, sheet or profile; and hotter at the die end to increase shear and mixing in the barrel. Extrusion dies can be much like those used for flexible PVC and are streamlined with land lengths 10-15 times the die opening. The take-up equipment is usually longer than that used for PVC with the profile passing through a warm bath (70-90°F) to eliminate residual tack and blocking on wind-up. Vacuum sizers and internally cooled mandrels are not recommended because of the soft, tacky nature of the thermoplastic urethane melt. Sheet extrusion is best carried out with a coathanger manifold die with stock temperatures running higher than for shape extrusion. A standard three-roll stack with roll temperatures decreasing progressively from 120°F to 80°F is used for take-up. General processing conditions for the extrusion of Pellethanes® 2363 are summarized in Table 3.

Table 3. General Processing — Extrusion (2-½ in. Extruder).

Grade			2363-80A	2363-90A	2363-55D
Barrel:	Rear,	°F.	370	380	390
	Middle,	°F.	380	390	400
	Front	°F.	390	400	410
	Adapter,	°F.	390	400	410
	Die,	°F.	390	400	410
	Melt,	°F.	400-420	410-430	415-435
	Feed throat		Cooling	Cooling	Cooling

Blown film has been produced using a side-fed polyethylene type die. Problems attributable to the blocking, toughness, and elasticity of the 2363 materials require modification in the conventional blown film slitting and winding setup.

Injection molding is done on standard reciprocating screw injection molding machines equipped with general purpose screws with compression ratios of between 2.2:1 and 3:1 and anti-backflow valves to ensure packing the mold cavity. Two-and three-plate molds are being used with the molds cored for temperature control. Sprues should contain a cold slug well at the exit chamber of the bushing with the well incorporating a Z-type, ring, etc. puller. Round runners are preferred and should be generous in diameter. Most gate designs are suitable except that pinpoint gates are not recommended for large parts. Generally, screw speeds of 40-90 rpm are employed with minimal back pressure (25-100 psig). Low injection pressures are required to fill the cavity at slow to moderate injection speeds. Cycle times will be dependent on part design, thickness, size and the particular grade of 2363 resin, but are in the order of what is required for most thermoplastic elastomers. Typical injection molding conditions for these materials are listed in Table 4.

Table 4. General Processing — Injection Molding (3 oz. Press).

Grade			2363-80A	2363-90A	2363-55D
Barrel:	Rear,	°F.	400	410	420
	Front,	°F.	400	410	420
	Nozzle,	°F.	410	410	420
Mold, °F.			100	100	100
Melt, °F.			425	430	435
Pressures:	Injection, psig		1000	1200	1400
	Back, psig		50	50	50
Injection, sec./hold, sec.			3/7	3/7	3/7
Cool, sec.			20	20	20
Shot size, gms			37	37	37

Segmented polyurethane elastomer solutions are also commercially available. For example, Biomer is based on DuPont's Lycra formulation, and this product is available as a solution (30% solid content) in dimethylacetamide [4]. Film cast from this solution exhibits tensile strength of 4,000 to 5,000 psi with a flexural modulus of 1,800 psi. Biomer is also available in tubing form, reinforced with stainless steel wire. Biomer is essentially inert in living tissue, and it is relatively non-thrombogenic in vascular systems.

Another group of segmented polyurethane elastomers (Tecoflex HR) were especially developed for use in heart assist devices [5]. These materials have the advantage over Biomer that they can be fabricated by the liquid casting techniques.

The liquid polyurethane elastomer systems can be cast either by machine or by hand. With careful mixing and efficient degassing parts of up to 2000g can be cast by hand. A cast system consists of an A (iso-cyanate) and a B (polyol) component, and a catalyst. The catalyst can be incorporated into the B component, or it can be added to the B component prior to casting. Thorough mixing of both components is mandatory, and subsequent degassing is necessary to avoid bubble formation. The "pot life" of cast systems is designed to provide ample time for stirring and degassing. The reaction mixture is poured into a preheated mold (200-250°F) and allowed to cure in an oven at 250°F for about 30 minutes. A post cure after demolding (several hours at 250°F) produces optimal properties.

Typical polyurethane cast elastomer systems designed for use in biomedical applications include CPR X218-47-1 and CPR X218-48-1. These systems have a pot life of six minutes and gelation occurs after 10 minutes. Physical properties of the resultant elastomers before and after hydrolytic stability test (100% relative humidity at 158°F for one month) are shown in Table 5.

Table 5. Physical Properties of Typical Cast Elastomers Before and After Hydrolytic Stability Testing.

System Sample Physical Properties*	CPRX218-48-1 Before HST	X218-48-1 After Hydrolytic stability test	X218-47-1 Before HST	X218-47-1 After Hydrolytic stability test
Duro Hardness @ R.T.	55A	54A	75A	75-73A
Tensile strength, psi				
100% Modulus	217	112	623	572
200% Modulus	299	163	1018	957
300% Modulus	462	213	1542	1342
400% Modulus	703(1 sample)	268	2253	1757
500% Modulus	–	339	–	2282
Ultimate	749	572	2394	2491
Elongation, %	391	763	400	533
Elongation Set @ Break, %	2	30	4	40
Tear strength, Die C, pli	121	107	236	321
Tear strength, Split pli	11	18.7	28.3	55.5

*To serve only as a guide for engineering design. Values shown are average values obtained from laboratory specimens.

Avcothane 51 is an elastomeric copolymer based on 90% poly(ether urethane) and 10% poly (dimethylsiloxane). It combines the excellent engineering properties of polyurethanes with a silicone-like surface [6]. Avcothane 51 has been clinically implanted in more than 30,000 intra aortic balloon pumps. This application requires excellent blood compatibility as well as good flex life because occasionally the device is applied for several weeks of continuous operation. The following physical properties have been reported for Avcothane 51 [6]. (Table 6).

Table 6. Physical Properties for Avcothane 51.

Density g/cc	1.09
Tensile Strength, psi	6200
Elongation at break, %	580
Hardness, Shore A	72
Graves Tear Resistance, lb./in.	490
Dielectric strength, volts/mil	1500

Also elastomers based on a nondiscoloring aliphatic diisocyanate (Hylene W) have been used in the restoration of facial features and in prosthetic applications intended to restore swallowing, chewing and speaking. Such a material has also been proposed for use in soft lens applications [7].

Soluble thermoplastic polyester elastomers (Estanes) had been used in the early stages of development of implant devices, but complete hydrolysis was observed after one year of implantation [8].

Flexible Polyurethane Foams

Flexible polyurethane foams are also produced by reactions of isocyanates and polyols. The most common isocyanate for flexible foam applications is tolylene diisocyanate (TDI). The polyols can be polyesters or polyethers and the foam products are generally blown using a combination of water and a halocarbon, such as trichlorofluoro methane. The polyether polyols are usually preferred because of low cost and better processing and the derived foams are also hydrolytically more stable. Because of their open cell structure, flexible foams are ideally suited for packaging materials and for absorbent type applications, such as disposable surgical drapes. Medical bandages, having an open celled polyurethane foam inner layer coated on one side with a moisture impermeable flexible film and on the other side with an adhesive layer have been described in the patent literature [9]. Water absorptive flexible urethane foam has also been proposed for diaper and sanitary napkin applications [10]. Open cell polyurethane foam is also being used in blood oxygenation. The polyurethane foam is impregnated with a silicone defoaming liquid to prevent froth formation in the oxygenation of blood.

Rigid Polyurethane Foam

Most rigid polyurethane foams are made from polymeric isocyanates (crude MDI) and high functionality, low molecular weight polyols. These foams are usually halocarbon blown and can be produced in densities ranging from 0.5-60 lbs./cu.ft. Because of their light weight and durability, rigid polyurethane foams have been used to replace wood in artificial legs and arms. They have also been used as casts for broken bones. For example, a liquid polyurethane foam system has been used to impregnate moist cotton cloth. The impregnated cloth is then attached to the body and curing of the foam occurs in approximately twenty minutes. A zipper can be incorporated into the cast for easy removal.

This system has been tested on several thousand patients [11]. The use of polyurethane foam (octamer) as a bone substitute has been described also, and it was recommended to use the foam in bone cysts and bone fracture repair. The foam was prepared from liquid components at the time of surgery [12].

CONCLUSION

Polyurethane is the polymer of choice for a wide variety of biomedical applications. The recent commercial availability of thermoplastic polyurethane elastomers suitable for medical and food applications has already prompted their use in the fabrication of hemodialysis sets, blood oxygenation tubing, i.v. sets, catheters, blood bags, solution containers, stoppers, endotracheal tubes, gas therapy tubing, heart assist devices, food conveyor belts and in a variety of other biomedical devices. Earlier results on experimental materials must be judged with caution because many of these materials were uncharacterized in terms of chemical composition, let alone trace effects of impurities. It is encouraging that heart assist devices formulated from polyurethane elastomer have shown the longest survival in calves [13,15]. Their flex endurance, wear resistance and vascular acceptability have made segmented polyurethane elastomers the materials of choice for heart assist pumps [14]. Attempts to produce non-clotting polyurethane implants for blood vessel, nerve, bile duct, ureter and bladder repair are continuing [15], and advances in fabrication as well as in the elucidation of structure and improvements in the methods for characterization of polyurethane elastomers have produced superior materials [16].

ACKNOWLEDGEMENTS

The authors wish to thank Mr. Bob Ward of AVCO Medical Products, Dr. David Wasserman of Ethicon and Mr. Mike Szycher of Thermo Electron Corporation for furnishing us with the technical data on Avcothane, Biomer and Tecoflex included in this paper.

REFERENCES

1.   G.C. Covolos, H.W. Bonk, and H. Ulrich, "Thermoplastic Polyurethane. An Alternative to PVC for Food and Medical Applications", presented at the National Technical Conference of the S.P.E., November 8–10, 1977, Denver, Colorado.

2.   J. Autian, "Toxicological Evaluation of Biomaterials: Primary Acute Toxicity Screening Program," *Artificial Organs, 1*, No. 1, August 1977, pp. 53-60.

3.   H.W. Bonk, A.A. Sardanopoli, H. Ulrich, and A.A.R. Sayigh, J. Elastoplastics, *3*, 157 (1971).

4.   Biomer is a Segmented Polyether polyurethane, available from Ethicon, Inc., Somerville, New Jersey, 08876.

5.   M. Szycher, V. Poirier and J. Keiser, Trans. Am. Soc. Artif. Organs, 1977, 116.

6.   R.S. Ward, Jr. and E. Nyilas, "Organometallic Polymers", p. 219-229, Academic Press, New York, 1978.

7.   E.A. Blair and D.E. Hudgin, U.S. Pat. 3,786,034 (1974); Chem. Abstr. *81*, 54470 (1974).

8.   W.S. Pierce, "Polymers in Medicine and Surgery", p. 263-286, Plenum Publ. Co., New York, 1975.

9.   J.L. Chen, Ger. Offen. 2,631,277 (1977); Chem. Abstr. *86*, 177356 (1977).

10.   H. Harada and Y. Shimodoi, Japan Kokai 7675,796 (1976); Chem. Abstr. *86*, 96027 (1977).

11.   The liquid system is available from Elastogran, Lemforde, Germany, a subsidiary of BASF.

12.   S.F. Hulbert and L.S. Bowman, "Polymers in Medicine and Surgery", p. 161-166, Plenum Publ. Co., New York, 1975.

13.   J.H. Lawson, D.B. Olsen, E. Hershgold, J. Kolff, K. Hadfield, and W.J. Kolff, Trans. Am. Soc. Artif. Organs 1975, 368; J.W. Boretos, W.S. Pierce, R.E. Baier, A.F. Leroy, and H.J. Donachy, J. Biomed. Mat. Res. 1975, 327.

14.   J.W. Boretos and W.S. Pierce, J. Biomed. Mat. Res. 1968, 121; R. van Noort, B. Norris, and M.M. Black, Plast. Med. Surg. Conf. 1975, 12.

15.   D.J. Lyman, W.J. Seare, Jr., D. Albo, Jr., S. Bergman, J. Lamb, L.C. Metcalf and K. Richards, Intern. J. Polymeric Mat., *5*, 211 (1977).

16.   G.L. Wilkes, "Polymers in Medicine and Surgery", p. 45-75, Plenum Publ. Co., New York, 1975.

THE USE OF SEGMENTED POLYURETHANE IN VENTRICULAR ASSIST DEVICES AND ARTIFICIAL HEARTS*

Winfred M. Phillips, DSc., Professor

College of Engineering

William S. Pierce, M.D., Professor
Gerson Rosenberg, Ph.D., Senior Project Associate
James H. Donachy, Fabrication Specialist

College of Medicine

The Pennsylvania State University
312 Mechanical Engineering
University Park, Pennsylvania 16802

ABSTRACT

Biomer, a segmented polyether polyurethane, has been used successfully as the blood contacting surface in artificial heart pumps and left ventricular assist devices. The material has the long fatigue life and high tensile strength required for this application. Moreover, fabrication techniques have been developed for molding the material with an extremely smooth blood contacting surface. In vivo experiments confirm that the material is biocompatible and that thromboembolic complications are minimal for highly washed blood surfaces. Total heart replacement experiments of durations to 100 days and long term left ventricular assist experiments in calves exceeding four months in duration have shown that the segmented polyurethane performs well. A left ventricular assist device with a blood surface of smooth segmented polyurethane has been used clinically with success.

*This work was supported by NIH-NHLBI Contract 1-RO1-HL-20356-01, PHS Career Award 5 KO4 HL 00085-4, NIH Grant No. 5 RO1 HL 13426-08 and NSF Grant ENG-76-23220.

KEY WORDS

Artificial Heart, Left Ventricular Assist, Segmented Polyurethane.

INTRODUCTION

The use of segmented polyurethane in biomedical devices has been prevalent in recent years due to the favorable characteristics of the material for this application and the improved techniques for fabrication. The material has an extremely long fatigue life and a durable non-biodegradable nature. Those polyurethanes fabricated under the trade names Avcothane® (Avco Everett) and Biomer® (Ethicon Corporation) have seen considerable use in left ventricular assist devices and artificial hearts [1,2,3]. Due to the current favorable experience with these materials, it is useful to outline the devices for which the material is primarily used, the fundamental properties of segmented polyurethane, the fabrication techniques of the material and the recent history of use of the material in animal implants and clinical applications.

In selecting a prosthetic material for cardiovascular applications, the primary concern is biocompatibility with blood. This must be coupled with long fatigue life for artificial heart pumps and assist devices. Determining the material strength and other fundamental properties of the material are important in such cases. The realistic constraints in blood pump and catheter applications, then, involve material strength, blood compatibility and biodegradation.

One can certainly agree at the outset with the recent comments by Bruck that internal blood contacting surfaces must be blood compatible in two fundamental ways [4]. Thrombotic events that lead to deposition, attachment and organized thrombus growth must be avoided. In addition, one must be concerned with avoiding the creation of thrombi that may, or may not, remain at the activation site. It is certainly clear that most prosthetic materials begin their tenure in vivo with the deposition of a protein layer. The subsequent activation of platelets and evidence of thrombosis is variable [5]. It is probable that these potential thrombosis problems depend on surface motion, surface activation energies and the general microstructure of the material surface as viewed by plasma and blood. Apparently, two approaches to the resolution or stabilization of the situation are possible. On the one hand, flocked or other relatively rough surfaces may be employed in an attempt to grow a pseudoendothelium. An alternative method employs smooth materials in an attempt to avoid any deposition, anchoring or growth. The Pennsylvania State University Artificial Heart program and others use the latter technique and employ a segmented polyether polyurethane as a durable, biocompatible, microscopically smooth blood-contacting surface [6,7].

The first references to the use of segmented polyurethane elastomer (Lycra®, Dupont) were given by Boretos and Pierce in 1967 at the National Institutes of Health [8]. At that time, they reported the use of this material in assist pump chambers and arterial cannulae. These researchers further suggested that numerous biomedical devices could be fabricated from the material including tubing, cannulae, catheters, pacemaker lead wiring insulation and heart valves. Subsequent to this initial suggestion, numerous applications of this type of material in medical devices has been reported [7]. The description of the material properties, fabrication techniques and hemodynamic characteristics given here have broad application. The focus and emphasis in this paper will be the use of segmented polyurethane in blood pumps.

MATERIAL PROPERTIES AND FABRICATION

Bulk Properties

The polyurethanes currently in use in our laboratories for blood compatible surface-contact materials are members of the Spandex fiber family initially trade-named Lycra® by DuPont. This material has a combination of characteristics that cannot be found in other elastomers that might be employed when a high flex life and long term blood compatibility are required.

The vast majority of blood pump designs and prototypes currently in use employ a moving, flexing, blood contacting surface. In our experience, most models successful in long term *in vivo* experiments have been pneumatically driven. The blood containing sac must be nonporous, effectively isolating the driving medium (gas) from the blood. The elastomer should offer little or no resistance to movement in order to minimize positive driving pressures and vacuum necessary for operation. While it is perhaps unrealistic to assume that there will be no surface deposition or minor surface changes under long term use, the material must not undergo observable biodegradation or mechanical property changes.

A segmented polyurethane such as Biomer can be described as a polyether elastomer with hard segments of urea and soft segments of polyether glycol connected by urethane linkages. This structure results in a high elastic modulus, resistance to flex fatigue, and excellent stability over long periods. The virgin polymer has a viscosity of 900 to 1500 poise at 25°C.

Long term cycling of molded samples of segmented polyurethane (Biomer) under repeated cycling at 100% elongation showed a stabilization of the stress after eight cycles [9]. Early tests on the material have shown similar mechanical characteristics after long term *in vivo* use as a blood pump. Recent tests in our laboratory using the material as blood sacs for left ventricular assist devices and total artificial hearts have shown no statistically significant reduction in tensile strength or flexibility after long term use in the biological environment. There is some variation in individual samples, but there seems to be no obvious degradation due to exposure to blood, gas or vacuum (Table 1). The results of all studies to date indicate that a carefully fabricated sac is reliable from a mechanical fatigue point of view when subjected to 100% elongation or less for long terms. In fact, most testing machines fail prior to the failure of the material under these conditions and special accelerated testing methods are needed to determine the true limitations of the material for use in this application. The elastomer can be formed into any desired shape and heat set. In all cases, the shapes thus formed show rapid recovery after being stretched and resist flexure fatigue.

Fabrication Technique

The special properties of Biomer present some fabrication difficulties that limit the production techniques that may be employed. The material does not lend itself to injection molding or extrusion techniques. The high solvent boiling point requires heating for complete solvent evaporation. Items have been successfully formed of the material by solution molding, drying to remove the solvent and heat setting to stabilize the shape. The local properties of products can be altered by thickness variation or impregnating with limited stretch materials.

The fabrication of seam free sacs for blood pumps as total artificial hearts or left ventricular assist devices is accomplished as follows. An

Table I. Mechanical Properties of Segmented Polyurethane

A. Samples

Date Tested	Test Sheet #	Polymer	# Samples	% Elongation/ Std.Dev.	Tensile Stress(PSI) Std. Dev. @ 100% Elongation	Tensile Stress(PSI) Std. Dev. @ Break
12/17/77	11-12-6A	I058B-II	6	638./24.	----	4730./440.
12/17/77	12-3-6A	I058B-II	8	657./39.	----	4580./500.
12/17/77	12-13-6B	I058B-II	14	669./33.	----	5040./580.
12/26/77	1-31-7B	J226B	5	647./48.	777./64.	5680./840.
1/25/78	3-29-7D	J226B	7	697./24.	622./63.	5060./810.
2/10/78	5-5-7E	J226B	11	664./31.	686./71.	5470./730.
2/10/78	5-12-7C	J226B	14	626./36.	636./82.	5270./550.
2/10/78	6-14-7E	K103B	15	638./17.	638./71.	5060./510.
2/10/78	9-22-7A	J230B	7	653./17.	658./28.	5150./500.
2/10/78	12-5-7	J230B	13	672./24.	662./58.	5040./580.

TABLE I (cont'd.)

B. Total Artificial Heart Angle Port Blood Bags

Bag #	Polymer #	Date Tested	# Samples	Left/Right	Time Used (Days)	% Elongation/Std.Dev.	Tensile Stress(PSI)/Std.Dev. @ 100% Elongation	@ Break
5-19-C	173D-II	---	4	L	11	842./35.	428./15.	5060./564.
7-28-7	K103B	3/17/78	8	L	100	681./34.	577./144.	5493./860.
R10-4-7A	J230B	3/17/78	8	R	100	710./22.	711./80.	6393./308.

C. Left Ventricular Assist Angle Port Blood Bags

Bag #	Polymer #	Date Tested	# Samples	Left/Right	Time Used (Days)	% Elongation/Std.Dev.	Tensile Stress(PSI)/Std.Dev. @ 100% Elongation	@ Break
4-5-6C	173D	---	8		77	775./23.	---	5580./606.
1-18-7	I058B-II	2/10/78	9		91	751./68.	703./54.	5607./550.
6-21-7B	K103B	2/10/78	9		68	670./57.	391./81.	5028./539.

aluminum mold is machined from a block which is split along the center line of the inlet and outlet ports. This hollowed mold is preheated to 80°C along with Epolene C10 mold wax (Eastman Chemical Products, Inc., Kingsport, Tenn.). The mold is filled with the hot Epolene and placed in a cold water bath. After partial cooling, excess Epolene is poured from the mold. Following further cooling, the Epolene form is removed from the mold, sanded and polished to remove bubbles and fine surface imperfections. The form is then cleaned with propanol and deionized water.

Following cleaning, the form remains under a laminar flow hood for all subsequent handling to maintain dust free conditions and humidity control. The Epolene is inspected and suitable samples are dipped in Dow Corning #236 air drying dispersion (Dow Corning, Midland, Michigan). The dispersion is allowed to dry for 12 hours and the form is inspected again. The dispersion gives a glossy and extremely smooth surface, covers minor surface imperfections and renders any remaining irregularities visible. If the form is acceptable, it is ready to be dipped for coating with the Biomer solution.

The Biomer solution, supplied by the Ethicon Corporation, is diluted with Di Methyl Acetamide, mixed well and allowed to stabilize overnight. The clean, dispersion-coated Epolene form is dipped 5 to 7 times in this solution with a one hour drying time between applications in a 140° to 160°F heated air flow. The final coated form is heated at 150 to 160°F for 24 hours. The Epolene mold is then crushed and removed from the polyurethane sac.

The dispersion boot is removed and the elastomer sac is heat set to stabilize the polymer. A section of the inlet tube is examined by scanning electron microscope. If the surface is acceptable and the sac is to be used for implantation, these results are retained for comparison with surfaces following *in vivo* service. In addition, tensile and fatigue test samples are prepared from the same stock of Biomer to be compared with test samples taken from the sac following termination of *in vivo* experiments.

A case and cap are machined of polycarbonate or, more recently, polysulfone. Ball or disc type inlet and outlet valves are employed. Metal valve components are fabricated of highly polished 316L double vacuum melt stainless steel, and silicone rubber balls or Delrin® (DuPont) discs are employed. The outlet valve housing is fabricated of highly polished polycarbonate or polysulfone. The assembled pump is shown in Figure 1. The dimensions and capacity of this unit are shown in Table 2.

Table II. Engineering and Performance Characteristics of 4 Ventricles employed for Long Term, Continuous Mechanical Circulatory Assistance

	Sac Pump	Longitudinal Tethered Sac Pump	Transverse Tethered Sac Pump	Angle Port Pump
Length (cm)	10.5	11.0	10.3	10.2
Width (cm)	9.5	10.1	12.5	9.5
Thickness (cm)	4.4	5.0	5.3	6.0
Capacity (ml)	170.0	188.0	148.0	140.0
Static Stroke (ml)	98.0	103.0	110.0	118.0
Dynamic Stroke (ml)	93.0	100.0	110.0	105.0
Dynamic Ejection Fraction (%)	66.0	53.0	74.0	75.0
Maximum Output (L/min)	11.5	11.5	12.0	12.0

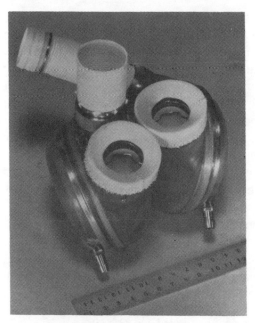

a. Total artificial heart pump.

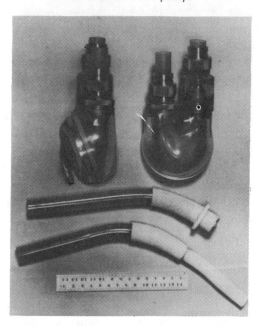

b. Left ventricular assist pump and cannulae

Figure 1. The Pennsylvania State University artificial heart.

The use of the blood pump as a left ventricular assist pump requires the fabrication of appropriate cannulae. The left ventricular cannula is fabricated by coating a silicone rubber dispersion-covered mandrel with Biomer. Certain areas are reinforced with a stainless steel wire wrapping. A final coat of polyurethane is used to cover the external surface of the wire. The arterial cannula is fabricated using a similar technique, except that a low porosity Dacron graft is connected to the distal end for anastomosis to the aorta. Obturators are fabricated using silicone rubber tubing. These obturators fit snugly within the left ventricular and aortic cannulae. A nylon tip on the obturator permits a firm attachment of tissue at the endocardial or endothelial surface.

Surface Properties

The favorable tensile and fatigue characteristics of segmented polyurethane allow concentration on the more critical question of blood-surface properties and behavior. It has been noted that the elastomer, Biomer, acquires a protein coating during long term exposure to blood [10]. This cell-free, polysaccharide-free, and lipid-free proteinaceous deposit seems to be a stable one that renders the surface passive to thrombus formation or embolization when the surface is subjected to dynamic blood contact. Phillips et al. [11] showed that a pump design resulting in effective surface washing is useful in maintaining this passive nature. The elastomer parts can be fabricated with extremely smooth surfaces that are resistant to water absorption (water absorption results in little change in tensile strength). Modified Lee-White clotting times performed in vitro with both canine and human blood compare favorably with results obtained with silicone rubber and are superior to Pyrex and siliconized glass [9].

Thick and thin films cast on smooth surfaces from commercial Biomer solutions have been shown to have surface tensions from 20 to 30 dynes/cm, relatively low values. In some cases, increased surface tension values and annealing-shifted contact angle values were observed indicating a lowering of the critical surface tension [10]. This result indicates that the fabrication of such segmented polyurethane elastomers must be done with care to avoid the formation of high energy surface structures generally assumed to adversely affect biocompatibility.

Detailed scanning electron microscope examinations of the Biomer surfaces prior to use and after long term implantation have been performed [12]. These studies show that extremely smooth surfaces can be fabricated and that there is little obvious correlation between the minor imperfections observed and cellular adhesion. There is some cellular material in some areas of the pump after long term implants but no animals exhibited signs of thromboembolism either clinically or post mortem.

IN VIVO **EXPERIENCE WITH SEGMENTED POLYURETHANE**

Left Ventricular Assistance

The left ventricular assist pump system consists of an inlet cannula from the left ventricle, the paracorporeally located blood pump (single ventricle), an outlet cannula to the aorta, a pneumatic power system and an electronic synchronization unit. Four different pump designs have been evaluated using Biomer as the blood contacting surface. In each case, a synchronization unit was used to control timing parameters of the power unit and was designed to trigger from the R-wave of the electrocardiogram. This automatic control system insured that the pump filled during cardiac systole and emptied during diastole.

The early design sac pump employed ball valves and a vacuum formed polycarbonate outer case. The pump specifications are given in Table 2. Flow visualization studies on a mock circulation system indicated that there was a low velocity region in the apex of this sac design [11]. A total of 536 days of continuous pumping with this device in 10 calves indicated that thrombus formation problems coincided with the poorly washed region. The pump required visual observation of the sac to permit optimal pumping without broad apposition of the sac walls. These problems resulted in a redesign of the blood pump.

The second generation pump design was a longitudinal tethered sac pump. This pump employed a flexible segmented polyurethane sac positioned within a rigid, cast epoxy case. A tether ring was attached to the outside of the sac, thus forming a pumping section similar to a seam free diaphragm pump. The dimension between the flexing member at end systole and the backside of the pump was controlled by proper positioning of the tether ring to prevent wall apposition. Ball-in-cage type inlet and outlet valves were employed. The specifications of this pump are shown in Table 2. A total of 243 days of continuous pumping was performed in 13 calves. Thromboembolic complications generally limited calf survival. Detailed flow visualization studies performed with this pump again indicated low flow velocity and poor washout in the apex area. Flow in this region was improved when Bjork-Shirley tilting disc type inlet valves were employed. However, disc or strut fractures have occurred in mock loop studies and the tilting disc valve was not employed in calf studies in a pump of this design. This pump was abandoned because of the low flow velocity in the apex and the high incidence of thrombi in that particular region.

The third pump evaluated was also fabricated of a smooth, flexible segmented polyurethane sac which was positioned in a molded polycarbonate case. In this instance, a flexible diaphragm served as a barrier between the apex of the sac and the molded polycarbonate case. This diaphragm limited the travel of the sac and prevented opposite wall contact. The size and output characteristics are shown in Table 2. Five calves underwent mechanical circulatory assistance for a total of 157 days. This pump had a considerably improved flow pattern in the apex area. However excessive sac stresses were present at the flexion line and in two calf experiments, sac tears occurred at this line. Use of this pump was discontinued because of the unacceptable sac stresses.

At this stage, certain facts regarding sac pump design become apparent. Sac washout and flow pattern appear to be of primary importance in preventing stasis and subsequent thrombus formation. The concept of adhering a portion of the sac to the case or of attaching a tether ring or other "appendage" to the external (nonblood-contacting) surface of the sac was unacceptable as thrombus occasionally adhered to the inner sac surface physiochemical structure of the polymer as a result of solvent or adhesive migration occurring. An angle port pump was designed to take advantage of this experience.

The angle port pump chamber is an ellipsoid having an elliptical cross section and a circular frontal section. The sac was designed to flex about the major circumference and to almost obliterate the blood space as seen on the cross sectional view. Because the maximum diameter of the inlet port was greater than one half of the thickness of the pump, it was necessary to place the ports at an angle to the ellipsoid. Thus, the sac motion was not restricted by the presence of the inlet or outlet ports as was the case in the longitudinal tethered sac pump. In order to prevent sac wall apposition, a diaphragm having a diameter equal to the circular frontal diameter of the pump has been placed between the cap and blood contacting sac. This diaphragm serves as a stroke limiter and prevents contaminants (i.e., grease, particulate matter) of the pneumatic power unit from contacting the external surface of the blood sac. An important feature of this pump is the ease with which the cap can be removed and an electrical energy converter-pusher plate combination attached to the pump. This conversion can be made from pneumatic to electrical power without design modification and without the need for an intermediate hydraulic converter.

The pump has undergone a variety of performance studies. Mock loop tests indicate a maximum flow rate of 15 liters per minute and a dynamic ejection fraction of 75% when ball valves are employed. Flow visualization studies indicate a good flow pattern with no stagnation at the apex area. The flow pattern and output are improved when tilting disc type inlet valves are employed. However, the mechanical durability of standard commercial tilting disc valves has not been satisfactory in all pneumatic blood pumps and ball valves have been employed in most of our animal implants.

This pump has now been employed for long term mechanical circulatory assistance in 11 calves. The total period of pumping in these calves has been 651 days with an average period of continuous pumping in each calf of 59 days. These calves have been treated with drugs to prevent platelet adhesion (aspirin and dipyrimadole) and the anticoagulant, warfarin sodium. There has been excellent maintenance of hemoglobin and hematocrit in these calves. The plasma hemoglobin has been in the range of 3 to 4 mg/dl. No abnormalities have been detected in the serum sodium, potassium, blood urea nitrogen, creatinine or bilirubin of these animals. In seven calves in this series, the left ventricular assist pump has been removed and the cannulae occluded with obturators. Each of these calves has been sacrified three (3) to eight (8) weeks later and a complete autopsy has been performed.

At the time of removal, the assist pump was generally clean, although in several calves a fine rim of fibrin was present along the flexion line. Scanning electron microscope studies of the sac showed occasional adherent platelets and subcellular debris. No tissue lining was present. Although there was no calf or clinical evidence of central nervous system emboli or renal emboli, a number of calves had small renol emboli at autopsy. The source of emboli in these heavily instrumented calves is not known and may be the pump, valves, or the left atrial or left ventricular pressure catheters. However, the relative freedom from thromboemboli in this pump design has been encouraging and the pump design continues to be used.

The angle port pump has also been employed in a series of calves in whom profound left ventricular failure has been produced by the intracoronary infusion of microspheres. The results are encouraging and indicate that initiation of assist pumping immediately restores aortic pressure to normal levels and concomitantly reduces left atrial pressure. Equally important is the observation that continued pumping has allowed an improvement in left ventricular function to occur over a time frame measured in days, permitting assist pump removal.

Total Artificial Heart

The segmented polyurethane material has been employed as the blood contacting surface in 26 total artificial heart experiments with calves [13]. The seamless segmented polyurethane sac is activated by a controlled air pulse introduced between the rigid polycarbonate case and the air diaphragm. The air pulse delivered by the drive system typically varies from a positive value for systolic ejection of approximately 220 mmHg to a diastolic vacuum of approximately − 30 mmHg. Wider variations in pressure are available as required. Each of the two ventricles employs two prosthetic valves and the appropriate Dacron connectors for suture. The pump can deliver up to 12 liters per minute with an ejection fraction of 75% and each ventricle is independently heat rate controlled by the automatic control system developed at The Pennsylvania State University [14]. This control system is employed to balance the output of the two ventricles, maintain physiologic pressures and increase cardiac output as required.

The blood pump design has evolved via *in vivo* testing for dynamic performance, flow characteristics and fatigue testing of the total prosthesis. Subsequent preliminary animal experiments were used to determine whether adequate cardiac output could be maintained in response to varying physiological needs; whether the operational mode, valves, connectors and general pump design were compatible with long term thrombus-free operation; and whether the pump and components could operate for long periods in the biological environmental without failure or degradation of performance, infection problems of other undesirable physiological difficulties (comfortable anatomical fit, pulmonary crowding as a function of change of position or exercise, etc.).

The latest total artificial heart design (the angle port pump) has been employed for both right and left ventricular replacement in six (6) calf experiments with survival times to 100 days. In all cases, the washed portions of the segmented polyurethane surface were thrombus-free. The first three (3) calves in this series all developed a linear tear in the blood sac after 60, 42 and 52 days of continuous pumping. A modification to the ventricle case relieved the high stress region and has eliminated the sac tearing problem. The next animal in the series lived 100 days. The cause of death was a disconnection of an improperly positioned atrial connector. The left atrial connector has since been modified to eliminate a subsequent occurrence of this problem. The last animal in this series lived 69 days and died of cerebral bleeding due to excessive anticoagulation.

The total artificial heart is a complex mechanical, material and physiological experiment and is a severe test of a biomaterial. The extensive blood contact is greater than in any other example and the segmented polyurethane performs well from a mechanical and thrombogenic viewpoint. The fabrication difficulties are far outweighed by the *in vivo* performance.

CLINICAL EXPERIENCE USING
MECHANICAL LEFT VENTRICULAR ASSISTANCE

A protocol to employ left ventricular assist pumping in patients with severe, refractory left ventricular failure was approved by the Clinical Investigation Committee of The Milton S. Hershey Medical Center of The Pennsylvania State University on August 15, 1976. An assist pump system and the necessary technical personnel have been available around the clock continuously since that time. The left ventricular assist pump has been employed in every patient operated upon since August, 1976 in whom the proper indications existed and in whom proper patient consent had been obtained. The results of this effort are summarized in Table 3. The first four (4) patients have been described in detail and will not be reiterated here (6). It is important to note that the third patient, S.F., who had required eight (8) days of continuous mechanical left ventricular assistance prior to pump removal, and cardiac cannulae obturation, continued to do well. She was able to perform the duties required of a farmer's wife and mother of four (4) children.

Table III. Summary of Clinical Experience – Mechanical Left Ventricular Assistance

Pt.	Age (Yrs)	Diagnosis	Operation	Emergency	Cardio-pulmonary Bypass Time (hrs)	Period of Left Ventricular Assistance (days)	Reason for Termination of Left Ventricular Assistance
NA	55	Mitral stenosis, severe pulmonary hypertension	Mitral valve replacement	No	$3\frac{1}{2}$	<1	Right ventricular failure secondary to severe pulmonary hypertension
IM	68	Aortic stenosis, cardiac arrest	Aortic valve replacement	Yes	$4\frac{1}{2}$	<1	Severe gastric bleeding
SF	39	Mitral	Mitral valve	No	$3\frac{1}{2}$	8	Good return of left ventricular function
RM	64	Aortic stenosis	Aortic valve replacement	Yes	$6\frac{1}{2}$	<1	Diffuse thoracic bleeding
MT	57	Left ventricular aneurysm	Resection of left ventricular aneurysm	No	$3\frac{1}{2}$	6	Good return of left ventricular function
CB	61	Left ventricular aneurysm	Resection of left ventricular aneurysm	Yes	$3\frac{1}{2}$	<1	Diffuse thoracic bleeding
CG	45	Mitral stenosis, aortic regurgitation	Mitral and aortic valve replacement	No	$2\frac{1}{2}$	<1	Primary right ventricular failure, poor assist pump filling

The fifth patient (M.T.) to require use of the assist device had undergone resection of a large left ventricular aneurysm and could not be weaned from cardiopulmonary bypass, even with the use of inotropic drugs and the intraaortic balloon pump. Use of the assist device subsequently allowed cardiopulmonary bypass to be discontinued. The patient had rather stable hemodynamic parameters during the six (6) days the assist pump was employed. The patient's left ventricular function progressively improved and supported the circulation well following pump removal. However, the patient's renal function deteriorated progressively from the time of the cardiac operation. The patient required renal dialysis and subsequently developed evidence of sepsis. The patient sustained multiple bouts of ventricular fibrillation and died 16 days after the cardiac operation (ten days following removal of the assist device). Pertinent autopsy findings were: (1) evidence of a recent myocardial infarction and (2) acute tubular necrosis of both kidneys with no evidence of renal emboli.

The sixth patient (C.B.) required emergency resection of a left ventricular aneurysm and could not be weaned from cardiopulmonary bypass. The assist pump was employed. However, pump filling was very poor and left atrial pressure remained low. When manual massage of the right ventricle was performed, or when inotropic drugs were employed, pump filling and arterial pressure improved. The hemodynamic condition finally stabilized with the use of dopamine hydrochloride to "support" the right ventricle and the assist pump to support the left ventricle. However, the patient had required an excessively long period of cardiopulmonary bypass and thoracic bleeding could not be controlled. This subsequently led to death of the patient.

The seventh patient (C.G.) had undergone double valve replacement and had a difficult first postoperative night. Twenty-four hours after operation, her systolic blood pressure was 80 mmHg, her cardiac index was 1 liter/min/m² and the heart was refractory to all pressor and inotropic drugs. The balloom pump was inserted but did little to improve the deteriorating cardiac status.

A subsequent cardiac index was 0.8 L/min/m². A decision was made to employ the assist device. The patient sustained a cardiac arrest on the way to the operating room. She was supported by external massage while the cannulae were inserted for cardiopulmonary bypass. The assist pump was inserted and pumping was begun. However, the pump filled poorly and the left atrial pressure remained low. The poor pump filling was a result of a right ventricular failure. Every possible attempt was employed to improve right ventricular output but the patient subsequently died.

Certain facts have become apparent in the course of this experience: (1) The smooth, seam free, segmented polyurethane paracorporeal assist pump is capable of supporting the entire systemic circulation of the adult human. Blood damage and thromboemboli do not represent serious problems. (2) Considerable cardiopulmonary bypass time is required to install the assist pump. Primary operation time, weaning effort and pump insertion time frequently result in excessive cardiopulmonary bypass time with an attendant risk of coagulopathy. Every effort must be made to simplify the insertion of the assist pump. (3) Proper positioning of the left ventricular cannula is of primary importance in obtaining high pump flow rates. The position of the cardiac apex when the chest is closed must be kept in mind during cannula insertion. A high left atrial pressure with poor pump filling suggests inlet cannula obstruction. (4) Primary right ventricular failure, due to poor cardiac muscle function, may result in poor pump filling. This problem can be isolated from inlet cannula obstruction by observing the left atrial pressure which remains low in right ventricular failure. Present information suggests that bilateral ventricular bypass will be required in order to provide proper cardiac support in certain patients. (5) We believe that an aggressive approach using mechanical left ventricular assistance should be continued. Improved results will occur when additional experience is gained, when techniques required to employ the device are simplified and when assist pumping is employed as promptly as possible when the proper indications exist.

REFERENCES

1. Pierce, W.S., "Polymers in Biomedical Devices: Materials for Artificial Heart and Circulatory Assist Devices", *Polymers in Medicine and Surgery* ed. R.L. Kronenthal, Z. Oser and E. Martin, Plenum Publishing Corp., New York, N.Y., pp. 263-285, 1975.
2. Boretos, J.W., Detmar, D.E. and Donachy, J.H., "Segmented Polyurethane: A Polyether Polymer, II. Two Years Experience", *J. Biomed. Mater. Res.* 5:373-387, 1971.
3. Lee, H. and Neville, K., *Handbook of Biomedical Plastics*, Pasadena Technology Press, pp. 6-1 — 6-96, 1971.
4. Bruck, S.D., "Biological Evaluation of Biomaterials for Cardiovascular Applications: Some Current Results", *Med. Prog. Technol.* 5:51-56, 1977.

5. Leonard, E.F., Butrille, Y., Puszkin, S. and Kochwa, S., "Blood Elements at Foreign Surfaces: Analysis of Inhomogeneities in Absorbed Layers of Proteins and Platelets", *Ann. N.Y. Acad. Sci. 283:256-269, 1977.*

6. Pierce, W.S., Donachy, J.H., Landis, D.L., et al., "Prolonged Support of the Left Ventricle", *Circulation,* Suppl. II, 1978 (In Press).

7. Jarvik, R.K., Lawson, J.H., Olsen, D.B., et al., "The Beat Goes On: Status of the Artificial Heart, 1977", *Int. J. Artificial Organs* 1 (1):21-27, 1978.

8. Boretos, J.W. and Pierce, W.S., "Segmented Polyurethane: A New Elastomer for Biomedical Applications", *Science* 158:1481, 1967.

9. Boretos, J.W., Pierce, W.S., Baier, R.E., Leroy, A.F. and Donachy, H.J., "Surface and Bulk Characteristics of a Polyether Urethane for Artificial Hearts", *J. Biomed. Mater. Res.* 9:327-340, 1975.

10. Baier, R.E., Personal communication.

11. Phillips, W.M., Brighton, J.A. and Pierce, W.S., "Artificial Heart Evaluation Using Flow Visualization Techniques," *Trans. ASME for Art. Int. Organs* 18:194-199, 1972.

12. Kurusz, M., Stover, L.R., Rosenberg, G., Donachy, J.H. and Pierce, W.S., "Scanning Electron Microscopy of Prosthetic Ventricles used for Left Ventricular Assist/Total Artificial Heart Devices: Preliminary Findings", *Proc. Workshop on Biomed. App.-SEM in Med. Prosthesis* 2: 221-228, 1977.

13. Pierce, W.S., Brighton, J.A., Donachy, J.H., Landis, D.L., Migliori, J.J., Prophet, A., White, W.J. and Waldhausen, J.A., "The Artificial Heart: Progress and Promise", *Arch. Surg.* 112:1430-1438, 1977.

14. Landis, D.L., Pierce, W.S., Rosenberg, G., Donachy, J.H. and Brighton, J.A., "Long Term *In Vivo* Automatic Electronic Control of the Artificial Heart", *Trans. Am. Soc. Art. Int. Organs* 23:519-524, 1977.

POLYOLEFIN BLOOD PUMP COMPONENTS*

Raymond J. Kiraly

Director of Engineering, Department of Artificial Organs
Cleveland Clinic Foundation
Cleveland, Ohio

Donald V. Hillegass

Research Chemist, Research Division
Goodyear Tire and Rubber Co.
Akron, Ohio

ABSTRACT

Implantable blood pump components are being fabricated from an EPDM type polymer, Hexsyn. This material has outstanding flex life and low toxicity and is stable. Blood pump diaphragms have been compression molded and evaluated extensively in vitro and in vivo. Good blood compatibility is achieved by impregnating glutaraldehyde crosslinked gelatin into a thin microporous layer formed in the rubber surface. Blood pumps containing these biolized diaphragms have been used up to 10.5 months in calves without anticoagulation.

KEY WORDS

Blood pumps, Diaphragms, High flex life, Polyolefin rubber, and Biolized surface.

*Work partially supported by NIH Contract NO1-HV-4-2960.

Material development specifically for cardiovascular applications has required polymers with high flex life and substantial blood compatibility. Our approach was to separate the requirements for mechanical properties from those requirements for blood compatibility. Our hypothesis regarding blood compatibility is based upon the good clinical results with aldehyde treated natural tissues in applications such as heart valves and vascular grafts [1]. Generally anticoagulants are not required with these materials. We coined the term "biolization" [2] to refer to aldehyde treated natural tissues and protein coatings both of which, we hypothesized, owe their blood compatibility to the crosslinked protein on the surface. Therefore, a material can be selected based on mechanical properties alone and then methods could be devised to obtain a biolized surface coating for blood compatibility. The search for a material with high flex life resulted in the development of Hexsyn, a polyolefin rubber [3], by the Goodyear Tire & Rubber Co. Hexsyn is an EPDM type of polymer prepared through solution polymerization. It has an interpolymer backbone of 1-hexene and methyl hexadiene and is crosslinked with sulfur.

HEXSYN PROPERTIES

For the past several years we have been exclusively utilizing this rubber for the pumping diaphragms [4] in both total hearts and assist pumps. Also other blood pump system components such as leaflet valves, stroke volume limiter diaphragms, and intrathoracic compliance bags have been molded from Hexsyn and used in various experiments. The flex life is being measured on a DeMattia test machine according to ASTM D-430, and after a remarkable 352 million cycles no damage was found. Table 1 compares the flex life of various polymers tested under identical conditions.

Over three years ago we initiated endurance testing of full-size Hexsyn diaphragms, both hemispherical and flat pusher-plate types. The diaphragms were pneumatically actuated through full stroke at a rate of 100 beats per minute submerged in 37°C saline. No flex failures in any of the rubber diaphragms has occurred with up to 146 million cycles accumulated. The outstanding flex life may be accounted for by several properties. First, it is a low modulus rubber which reduces interchain stress when the material is flexed. Secondly, its backbone is a straight

Table 1. Flex Life of Various Polymers ASTM D 430 De Mattia Test Machine.

Polymer	Cycles to Failure (millions)
Silicone rubber	0.8
styrene-butadiene rubber	4
natural rubber	4
oxypropylene rubber	10
Ethylene-propylene-diene-terpolymer	15
Biomer^R	18
Hexsyn	352 (no failure)

Table 2. Mechanical Properties of Hexsyn (Batch 7254-9).

Tensile strength, psi	1700
Elongation at break, %	450
100% Modulus, psi	210
300% Modulus, psi ASTM D412	970
Crescent Tear, pli ASTM D624	180
Instron Tear, pli	4.9
Tension set, % @ 100% elongation ASTM D412	5

chain saturated hydrocarbon totally resistant to oxidation and ozonation, thereby eliminating the oxidative erosion that normally occurs in surface imperfections on conventional, unsaturated rubbers. It is a sulfur vulcanized compound, and its viscosity allows compression, injection, or transfer molding in manufacturing the required product. Extraneous sulfur and other processing agents are removed following vulcanization by extraction with acetone and toluene, leaving a pure hydrocarbon polymer with excellent physical and chemical properties. Table 2 lists some of the mechanical properties of a representative batch of Hexsyn rubber. Hydrolysis aging tests showed that the rubber's properties were unaltered after 120 days at 70°C and 100% relative humidity. It is also significant that tensile tests performed on specimens cut from blood pump diaphragms used in vivo, including a total artificial heart implanted for 145 days and an assist pump implanted for 316 days showed that the mechanical properties were not markedly changed from those shown in Table 2. Samples of Hexsyn rubber are being provided to NHLBI Devices and Technology Branch contractors for independent evaluation of physical and mechanical properties, especially those relevant to long-term blood pump diaphragm applications. Since these contractors are currently developing meaningful test procedures, specific comparative data should be available soon.

In order to evaluate the toxicity of Hexsyn rubber, samples were compression molded into sheets, cleaned, and sterilized according to the same procedures used in preparing diaphragms for assembly into blood pumps. The sample sheets were sent to the Material Science Toxicology Laboratories at the University of Tennessee for toxicity testing. A complete test series [5] was conducted for biological evaluation including tissue culture agar overlay, rabbit muscle implants, hemolysis testing, systemic toxicity and cell growth inhibition. All tests were negative except for the tissue culture agar overlay which showed the lowest level of detectable toxicity. The University of Tennessee concluded that Hexsyn had a very low order of toxicity. Also subsequent to these evaluations, the solvent extraction procedures were improved for more effective removal of residual processing components from the rubber to further reduce toxicity.

Water vapor transmission, an important consideration for a long-term implant of a closed system, was evaluated by test methods specified in ASTM E-96. Hexsyn compression molded sheets, nominally 1.0 mm in thickness were tested at 35°C. The permeability was 6.0×10^{-3} g/24 hr-m^2-mmHg/cm thickness.

DIAPHRAGM FABRICATION

Table 3. Hexsyn Rubber Formulation.

Constituent	Concentration
Polymer	100.0
ISAF Black	50.0
Zinc Oxide	2.0
Stearic Acid	2.0
Tetramethyl thiuram disulfide	1.0
2-Mercaptobenzothiazole	0.5
Sulfur	2.0

Table 3 lists the constituents in the rubber used in the diaphragms. Compounding and mixing procedures are as outlined in ASTM Designation D 3182. A BR Banbury internal mixer is used for mixing the base polymer, pigment, and accelerator activators. The mix is batched off onto an 8″ × 16″ mill and then transferred to a 6″ × 16″ laboratory mill for addition of the accelerators and the vulcanization agent. To minimize particulate contamination the mixing surfaces of the equipment are blown with an air jet. The batch is also preceded through the mixing operation by a pure batch of natural rubber to further clean the equipment. All subsequent fabrication steps are done within a laminar flow clean air work bench to minimize particulate contamination.

Figure 1 is a photograph of two compression molds used to fabricate two different pump diaphragms. The molding procedure consists of adding a preweighed amount of the compounded rubber to the mold preheated to 310°F. The mold is closed and placed into a hydraulic press. A load of 30,000 lbs is applied for 10 minutes. The 10 minutes represents enough cure to allow some sulfur crosslinking and sufficient substance to the diaphragm for removal from the mold and application of the textured blood contact surface. A typical Rheometer curve for the

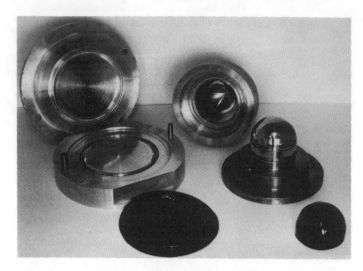

Figure 1. Compression molds and produced rubber diaphragms.
Flat 4-inch diameter diaphragm on left is for use in parathoracic
pusher plate pump. Hemispherical diaphragm on right is for the
pneumatically driven intrathoracic LVAD. Virtually any shape
diaphragm or component can be compression molded.

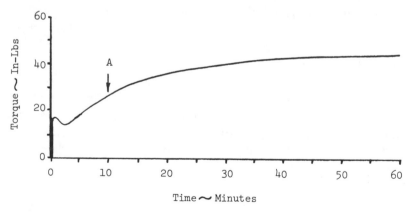

Figure 2. Rheometer cure curve for 60 minutes at 310°F showing typical polyolefin
cure behavior. Point A represents end of partial cure. (ASTM D 2084-75).

material under curing conditions is shown in Figure 2. Point A represents
the time during cure at which the diaphragm is removed from the mold.
After the mold is removed from the press and opened, the partially cured

diaphragm is removed, visually inspected, and prepared for surface texturing. The purpose of the textured surface is to mechanically hold the biolized coating (aldehyde treated gelatin) for blood compatibility. The porous surface is formed integral with the rubber surface by a salt casting technique. Reagent grade sodium chloride is pulverized in a Waring blender and mechanically graded to obtain salt particles passing through a 250 micron sieve and retained on a 109 micron sieve. This salt is mixed with an equal weight of solution made up of 10% by weight of rubber dissolved in toluene. After compression molding of the diaphragm, but prior to complete curing, three coats of the salt-rubber mixture is painted on the blood contacting surface. The diaphragm with the salt-rubber coating is then vacuum dried to evaporate the solvent. Final oven curing of the diaphragm causes the texture to become integrally bonded to the substrate rubber. Subsequent to curing of the rubber, the diaphragm is rinsed in water to dissolve the salt remaining with the pores. This sequence is shown schematically in Figure 3. Figure 4 is a scanning electron micrograph of the textured surface formed by this method. The thickness of the porous layer is approximately 100 microns and the pore size is in the range of 10 to 50 microns.

The diaphragm is again carefully inspected for surface flaws and then solvent extracted in a 70% acetone, 30% toluene mixture for six hours to remove excess accelerator and residual sulfur from the rubber. The diaphragms are then vacuum dried and submerged in boiling water for one hour to remove all residual solvent.

DIAPHRAGM BIOLIZATION

Biolization is accomplished by aldehyde treating a gelatin coating impregnated into the textured surface on the blood contact side of the diaphragms. Eastman Kodak 1099 gelatin was used initially, but when that product became unavailable it was replaced by Fisher G-7. There was no observable difference in the performance of these two gelatins, particularly in in vivo blood compatibility in calf-implanted pumps. Mechanical properties of several different gelatins are currently under study including effects of variations in the coating procedures. The mechanical properties of the crosslinked gelatin are important when the stress and strain induced by the flexing diaphragm are considered. Although these studies are continuing, it appears that the present procedures are adequate but it is not known whether they are optimum.

SALT CAST TECHNIQUE FOR TEXTURING SURFACE

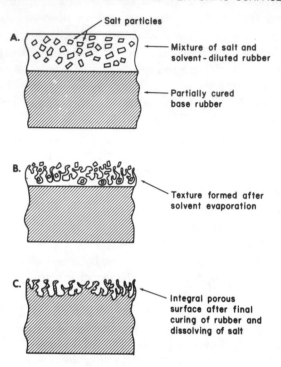

Figure 3. Method used to produce 100 micron thick porous textured surface integral with the diaphragm. Surface is subsequently biolized by filling pores with glutaraldehyde treated gelatin.

Five percent by weight of gelatin is dissolved in deionized water at 60°C and the solution is then degassed under vacuum. The diaphragm is then submerged in the warm solution and placed in a vacuum oven. The oven is evacuated for 30 minutes and returned to atmospheric for five minutes followed by a second evacuation for five minutes and returned to atmospheric pressure and to assure complete air removal and gelatin impregnation into the pores. The diaphragm is then removed from the solution and placed into a humidified chamber at 4°C for 15 minutes to gel the coating. The diaphragm is then removed and dipped into the gelatin solution for a few seconds and then returned to the cold chamber for an additional 15 minutes. This dipping and gelling process is then repeated. The diaphragm is then immersed into a 0.45% buffered glutaraldehyde solution at 4°C for 12 hours for crosslinking [7].

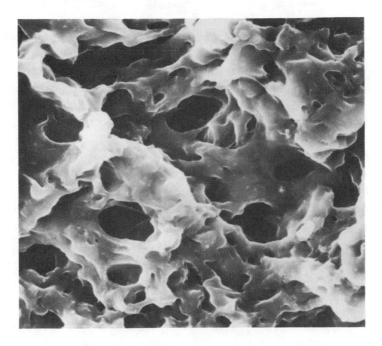

Figure 4. SEM (1000X, 1.0 cm = 10 microns) of textured surface produced on diaphragm surface. Pore sizes range between 10 and 50 microns.

It was found to be absolutely essential that the gelatin solution layer be gelled prior to aldehyde treatment in order to have a stable, consistent well crosslinked coating. Gelation of the 5% Fisher gelatin solution occurs between 15 and 20°C. In a previous method [4] the gelatin was brushed onto the diaphragm at room temperature. Then the diaphragm was submerged in glutaraldehyde for one day at room temperature. By using this method some diaphragms were clean without any macroscopical deposition even after 59 days of in vivo use. The results however were inconsistent and scanning electron microscopical study of these diaphragms showed instances of 1) cracks and/or detachment of gelatin layer, 2) inconsistent thickness of the gelatin layer on top of the textured rubber and 3) poor impregnation of gelatin into the textured layer [6]. To overcome these problems, the above described current method was developed. By applying vacuum while the diaphragm is submerged in the gelatin solution, the gelatin completely fills and covers the porous rubber, resulting in a continuous smooth gelatin blood contact surface.

It should be pointed out that by varying the gelatin concentration in the coating procedure, different degrees of surface covering can be achieved. In this way some surface texture or porosity can be retained, while the gelatin progressively fills larger and larger pores as the concentration is increased. The present 5% gelatin coating completely covers the texture, but if some texture is desired, for example to simulate flocked surfaces, then this can be obtained by appropriately lowering the gelatin concentration in the processing.

The mechanical characteristics of the gelatin coated diaphragms were examined using a Scott-CRE/500 tensile tester. All testing was done at room temperature with special attention paid to the cracking of the gelatin layer. The dumbbell-shaped rubber samples were gelatin coated and glutaraldehyde treated according to the most recent procedure. The gelatin coating on the textured surface did not appreciably change the stress-strain characteristics of the base rubber material.

As the extension of specimen increased, faint streaks appeared initially and definite cracks occurred later only in the gelatin layer. The streaks initially occurred at about 20% extension of the rubber with cracks appearing at 60% extension of the rubber. From this result, a maximum elongation of 15% is designed into diaphragms for blood pumps under development. Studies are now underway to determine the effect of coating procedures on the mechanical properties of the gelatin coating on the rubber. It may be possible to obtain a more elastic gelatin coating on the diaphragm for an added factor of safety in design.

Samples of biolized Hexsyn have been supplied to several biomaterials researchers for evaluation [8]. Although the results are not available as of this writing, publication of the various tests and results are expected in the near future. Also, up to the present time, gelatin has been the only protein used for diaphragm biolization. Other proteins, however, such as albumin, fibrinogen and fibrin, and collagen may have advantages over gelatin and are being studied as well.

DIAPHRAGM IN VIVO RESULTS

The results of different degrees of gelatin coating of the porous rubber were evaluated [9]. The 5% coating completely covers over the porous surface, while a thinner 1% solution coats and fills some of the smaller pores, leaving the larger pores open and retaining the general surface texture. Biolized total hearts and assist pumps using these diaphragms were implanted in 90 Kg calves without postoperative anticoagulants. In experiments of over one week duration, 5% gelation coatings were used in 14 total heart experiments of up to 145 days, and 11 assist pumps of up to 316 days; 1% gelatin coatings were used in three total heart experiments of up to 94 days and six assist pump experiments of up to 210 days.

The pseudoneointima (PNI) formed on the diaphragms coated with 1% gelatin appeared similar to that observed on fabric covered [10] or flocked surfaces, being of variable thickess largely dependent upon the local blood flow conditions. After one day, a thin whitish deposit, especially at the periphery, is seen composed of a platelet-fibrin matrix with various degrees of white and red cell entrapment. Fibroblast invasion was not observed even after 99 days of implantation with PNI thickness up to 3mm and generally thickest at the diaphragm-housing junction. When systemic infection occurred, bacterial colonization was found in the thicker, nonstabilized PNI.

In contrast, the 5% gelation coated diaphragms were generally free of any measurable deposition where the gelatin completely covered over the rubber and remained intact. Coatings applied by brushing showed a definite continuous layer of gelatin on top of the textured rubber although the gelatin was not well impregnated into the porous structure. Insular depositions were frequently observed although the majority of the surface remained smooth and clean. It was clearly documented that deposition occurred in the local areas where the gelatin had detached from the surface.

The "vacuum dripping" method of coating was successful in completely filling the porous network of the rubber which should result in better mechanical anchoring of the gelatin coating. Even with this method, cases where the gelatin layer was not completely gelled prior to aldehyde treatment resulted in a brittle coating which easily cracked and detached during diaphragm flexing. These cases also resulted in localized deposition over the defects. It should be remembered that the results described here are for hemispherical diaphragms which have relatively uncontrolled surface motion during flexing resulting in possible local high strain areas contributing to overstressing the gelatin coating and consequent cracking and detachment. Pusher plate pump diaphragm motion can generally be controlled and designed for low deformation to avoid damage to the gelatin coating. This was done in the case of the design of an intrathoracic pusher plate pump [6] currently under development with an adequate safety margin in the deformation of the gelatin coated diaphragm.

In pumps where reasonable blood flows were maintained for the entire experimental period, the 5% gelatin-coated diaphragms generally retained the original gelatin coating which appeared smooth and glistening, covering over the rubber surface with no macroscopic deposition observable. When observed by higher magnification, it was shown that the gelatin surface is covered by a proteinaceous material and the blood corpuscles attaching to it are not morphologically activated. The platelets were either a "contact" type or a "spread" type in shape, but aggregation formation was not observed. It is interesting that the flattened cells were observed on the 5% gelatin surface as early as two weeks of implantation. These findings suggest that the glutaraldehyde treated gelatin "smooth" surface is quite blood compatible. The nature and origin of the flattened cells are not known yet; however, they seem to be very similar to the flattened endothelial-like cells found in the pericardium lining of the pump housing which were shown to be the precursor cells of endothelial cells [11].

CONCLUSIONS

A high-flex life rubber, Hexsyn, has been successfully used in blood pump components and has particular advantage for long-term implantation. The excellent mechanical properties are complemented by good blood compatibility achieved by incorporating an aldehyde-crosslinked gelatin coating impregnated into the porous surface of the rubber. While development and optimization continues, it appears that Hexsyn and the biolized blood contact surface can adequately meet blood pump diaphragm requirements.

REFERENCES

1.   R.J. Kiraly and Y. Nose, Natural tissue as a biomaterial. Biomat, Med. Dev, Artif Organs, 2:207, 1974.

2.   Y. Nose, K. Tajima, Y. Imai, M. Klain, G. Mrava, K. Schriber, K. Urbanek and H. Ogawa. Artificial heart constructed with biological material. Trans Am Soc Artif Intern Organs, 17:482, 1971.

3. J. Lal and P.H. Sandstrom. Sulfur Vulcanizable Interpolymers. U.S. Patent 3,933,769, January 20, 1976.
4. R.J. Kiraly, R. Arconti, D. Hillegass, H. Harasaki and Y. Nose. High flex rubber for blood pump diaphragms. Trans Am Soc Artif Intern Organs 23:127, 1977.
5. E.O. Dillingham, N. Webb, W.H. Lawrence and J. Autian. Biological evaluation of polymers. 1. Poly(methyl methacrylate). J. Biomed. Mater Res, 9:569, 1975.
6. Development and Evaluation of Cardiac Prostheses. Annual Report NO1-HV-4-2960-4. Y. Nose, Principal Investigator. June, 1978.
7. H. Kambic, G. Picha, R. Kiraly, I. Koshino and Y. Nose. Application of aldehyde treatments to cardiovascular devices. Trans Am Soc Artif Intern Organs, 22:664, 1976.
8. R.J. Kiraly, Y. Nose and H. Kambic. Biolized materials. Devices and Technology Branch Contractors Conference Proceedings, 1977, pg. 166.
9. H. Harasaki, R.J. Kiraly, D. Hillegass, H. Kambic and Y. Nose. Evaluation of biolized blood pump diaphragms. Trans 4th Annual Meeting Society for Biomaterials & 10th Annual International Biomaterials Symposium 1978, pg. 105.
10. G. Picha, M. Helmus, S. Barenberg, D. Gibbons, R. Martin and Y. Nose. The characterization of intima development in left ventricular assist device (LVAD) and total artificial heart (TAH). Trans Am Soc Artif Intern Organs, 22:554, 1976.
11. H. Harasaki, R. Kiraly and Y. Nose. Endothelialization in blood pumps. Trans Am Soc Artif Intern Organs, 24:415, 1978.

FABRICATION AND TESTING
OF FLOCKED BLOOD PUMP BLADDERS

Victor Poirier

*Thermo Electron Corporation
Research and Development Center
Biomedical Systems Department
45 First Avenue
Waltham, Massachusetts 02154*

Thermo Electron Corporation has been involved in the development and fabrication of blood pumps and heart assist components for the last 15 years. During this time period, many devices and components have been evaluated in order to arrive at a unit capable of being utilized in the clinical arena. Figure 1 illustrates such a blood pump.

As shown, the pump consists of a flexible bladder fabricated from polyurethane. This bladder, positioned inside a titanium housing, forms the main pumping chamber. Programmed pneumatic pulses enter the void volume between the bladder and the metallic housing to deform the bladder in a three-lobe fashion, expelling 75 ml of blood volume. The bladder, 5.2 cm in diameter by 8.7 cm in length, is positioned between blood-carrying conduits, fabricated from rigid metal members, and flexible Dacron graft. At the extreme end of the inlet conduit is positioned a titanium tube that is ultimately inserted into the apex of the left ventricle. Attached to this inlet tube is the inlet valve designed to permit only unidirectional flow. This porcine xenograft valve is sutured directly to the vascular graft, which is protected by a Silastic conduit. The outlet conduit is similarly constructed and is anastomosed to the ascending aorta to complete the connection to the vascular system. All blood-contacting surfaces, except the vascular graft and valves, are coated with polyester fibrils to form an appropriate anchoring mechanism for the formation of an antithrombogenic biologic surface.

Supported in part by the NHLBI under the following contracts: NO1-HI-4-2910; NO1-HV-2915; NO1-HV-5-308; NO1-HV-7-2976- NO1-HV-7-2934; NO1-HV-7-2936; NO1-2907; NO1-HV-3-2946; NO1-HL-2065.

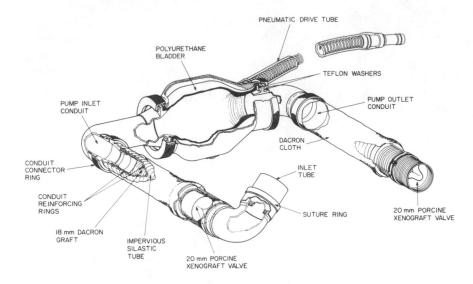

Figure 1. Model 10 Temporary Left Ventricular Assist Device.

The bladder utilized in this device must be capable of undergoing severe service if it is to replace the nonfunctioning biologic left heart. Therefore, it must be able to flex at least 40×10^6 cycles per year and withstand the hostile environment of the body without significant degradation, and must be biologically acceptable and nontoxic.

To achieve these goals, several materials and coating processes were evaluated. Initially, commercially available elastomers were used because materials had not been developed specifically for this application. Gradually, however, better materials became available — first, silicone elastomers and, later, urethane polymers. These also were evaluated, and each proved to be superior to its predecessor.

A similar evaluation process was used for blood interface surfaces. Initially, smooth surfaces were evaluated, then electrically charged surfaces, and finally rough-textured fibril surfaces. Again, each successive step was an improvement over the previous one.

BLADDER MATERIALS AND FABRICATION TECHNIQUES

Silicone Elastomer (Dow Corning)

In the fabrication of implantable prostheses, care must be taken to ensure that the material is of medical grade. Dow Corning's Silastic [1] meets this requirement. These silicone rubber compounds are prepared in medical manufacturing facilities that assure an environment of minimum contamination. All compounding and handling is done in a filtered-air atmosphere, and all personnel are clad in lint-free clothing. The compounds are graded as soft (MDX 4-4512, 25 shore A), medium (MDX 4-4515, 50 shore A), and firm (MDX 4-4516, 75 shore A).

Two types of silicone polymers, both of which are predominantly polydimethylsiloxane, are used in formulating Dow Corning's Clean-Grade Elastomers. The medium and hard grades are made from polydimethylsiloxane copolymerized with small amounts of methylvinylsiloxane. This particular copolymer makes for a more efficient vulcanization, and yields a rubber that has the properties shown in Table 1. The soft grade is made from a copolymer of dimethylsiloxane, and methylvinylsiloxane that contains a small portion of phenylmethylsilox-ane whose presence contributes to the softness of the rubber.

Table 1. Clean Room Grade Silastic (Dow Corning).

Property	Soft Grade MDX4-4514	Medium Grade MDX4-4515	Firm Grade MDX4-4516
Color	Clear Translucent	Clear Translucent	Clear Translucent
Specific Gravity	1.12	1.14	1.23
Durometer Hardness Shore A	25	50	75
Tensile Strength, psi	850	1200	1000
Elongation, %	600	450	350

A filler of fine silica particles is used in these three grades of Silastic. These small and amorphous particles interact with the polymer molecule to reinforce the rubber. Dichlorobenzoyl peroxide, an unstable peroxide used as the vulcanizing agent in this material, decomposes when heated, and initiates a free radical reaction that forms cross-linkages between adjacent polymer chains.

The vulcanized silicone rubber is soft, putty-like material that lends itself to easy handling and fabrication by conventional rubber fabricating techniques, such as molding, extruding, and calendering. The material is available in sheets that are one foot square and varys in thickness from 0.25 mm and up. Dacron mesh can be added to provide additional strength from 0.5 mm and up.

Bladders fabricated from this material have operated for an excess of 25×10^6 cycles without failure [2]. In addition, the fabricated material can be readily steam sterilized without causing appreciable changes in the physical or chemical properties. Also, the material is extremely well tolerated by the body [3] and is, therefore, very suitable for use in implantable devices.

In summary, the first silicone rubber compounded specifically for medical purposes was produced in 1953. Since that time, a vast number of implantable devices have been constructed from this material and utilized in patients. The advantages and disadvantages of the material are listed for the reader's information.

Advantages
- It is easily fabricated.
- It is biocompatible.
- It is elastomeric.
- It can be sterilized in steam.
- It is resistant to aging.
- It is nonadhesive.
- It is reinforcible with Dacron mesh.
- It is available as medical grade.
- It is permeable to gas and water vapor.
- It is chemically resistant.

Disadvantages
- It has a limited flex life.
- It is permeable to water vapor.
- It is difficult to flock.
- It is distorted by liquid absorption.
- It has a low tensile strength of 850 to 1200 psi at 350- to 600-percent elongation.

Silastic Fabrication

Two fabrication techniques have been developed to manufacture Silastic blood-pump components. The first, compression molding, is used to fabricate reproducible components after a design has been established. The second, "hand lay-up," is used to fabricate prototype components that are undergoing continuous change.

Compression Molding

A hydraulic press, shown in Figure 2, and an appropriately designed mold, shown in Figure 3, are necessary to fabricate components by the compression molding technique. The press, or mold, must be capable of being heat cycled to 145°C, and subsequently water cooled to room temperature. Depending on the size of the component, the press should also be capable of producing up to a 50-ton load.

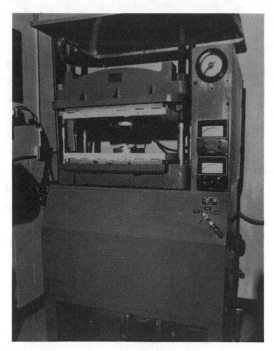

Figure 2. 50-Ton hydraulic press.

The mold should be fabricated from aluminum to allow for rapid temperature changes and uniform heat distribution. The design must provide sufficient surface area on the mold bearing surfaces to transfer the 50-ton load without yielding the aluminum. A release agent must be used on the surfaces that will be exposed to the Silastic. Teflon coating or mold release agent can be used. If Teflon coating is used, the mold must be designed with larger bearing surfaces in that the aluminum will be annealed during the coating process and thus reduced in strength.

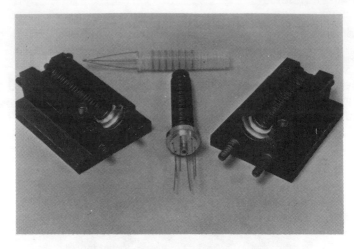

Figure 3. Silastic compression mold.

In order to accommodate Silastic shrinkage during processing, the mold is designed to be 1.5 percent larger than the component being fabricated. Also, the design should provide release ports (0.2 mm high × 0.5 cm wide) in the mold to allow for overflow of excess Silastic. These should be positioned as far away from the Silastic loading site as possible.

The mold is designed to be split at a noncrucial point of the component. One half is mounted to the top platten and the other to the bottom platten of the hydraulic press. These plattens are equipped with water cooling channels and heaters, which are used to control mold temperatures. Alignment guide pins in the mold proper provide the exact alignment required for precision parts.

Several trial runs are necessary to determine the amount of Silastic required. Once this has been established, the mold can be loaded with the proper weight of uncured Silastic (MDX 4-4515). Care must be taken to ensure that the mold is scrupulously cleaned and handled only with polyethylene gloves. After loading, the mold is closed, pressure applied, and the Silastic is allowed to overflow through the release ports. The mold is then heated to 116°C for 30 min. This temperature crosslinks the Silastic on the mold so that it can be easily removed after cooling. The fabricated diaphragm is removed, boiled in soapy water (Ivory Snow) for 30 min, flushed with distilled water, and then boiled two additional times for 30 min each. The component is then post-cured for 3 hr at 150°C in an air-circulating oven. Since component geometry strongly influences temperature cycling time, trial runs for every new mold are necessary to establish the proper processing cycles. Once established, they are reproducible and can be well controlled.

The compression molding technique can be used to fabricate complex geometries in a reproducible manner. It has the added flexibility of allowing the insertion of metal or plastic components to fabricate assemblies with multiple parts. These can be molded directly into the Silastic components or added after vulcanization with adhesives such as Dow Corning's Medical-Grade Adhesive 891. Figure 4 illustrates some typical components that have been fabricated by this process and used as implantable devices.

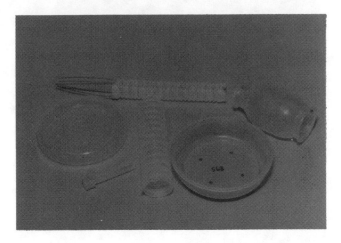

Figure 4. Typical compression-molded components of silastic.

Hand Lay-Up

The hand lay-up technique is a very flexible fabrication technique used to build prototype components or components that must be reinforced with Dacron mesh. Dow Corning uncured Silastic (MDX 4-4515) is supplied in sheets of various thicknesses, with or without Dacron mesh. This sheeting, usually 1 mm thick, is applied to a mandrel machined to be 1.5 percent larger than the required finish dimensions. The mandrel, coated with Teflon or release agent, is positioned to receive the Silastic sheeting. This sheeting, with the protective plastic coating removed from one side, is placed on the mandrel and then rolled with a stainless steel buffed rolling tool to conform to the mandrel. It is necessary to apply a uniform rolling action along the entire mandrel surface in order to prevent and avoid air pockets and bubbles. Once the sheeting is in intimate contact with the mandrel, an 1/8-in. overlap is made at any intersection point to provide for a fused joint. The excess Silastic is trimmed off and the outer covering is removed. Critical areas can be reinforced by adding additional layers of Dacron reinforcing, or built-up with Adhesive 891.

The completed assembly is placed in an air-circulating oven and the Silastic is cured at 150°C for 3 hr. The component is then removed and washed as previously stated. Figure 5 illustrates components that have been fabricated by this technique.

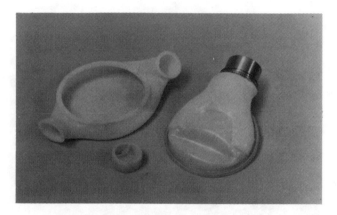

*Figure 5. Components fabricated from the
"Hand Layed Up" technique.*

It should be noted that sprayed-on mold release agents should be used only for experimental purposes since silicones are considered to be surface contaminants which can be impregnated during the process. Established mold designs should utilize permanent Teflon coatings.

Tecothane B (Thermo Electron)

Tecothane B is a two-component, polyester-based, cross-linked urethane. It is formulated by curing a reactive resin mixture of cyanaprene A-8 (American Cyanamid) and a specially formulated curative.

The curative consists of two active ingredients (crosslinker and catalyst) and an inactive carrier. The so-called crosslinker which reacts with the resin to form a polymer network, is trimethylolpropane (TMP). The other active ingredient is a tertiary amine, triethylene-diamine (Dabco), which influences the speed of reaction and the specificity of the chemical reactions. The amine, of course, does not become an integral part of the polymer.

The carrier, dimethyoxytetraethylene glycol, is a solvent for TMP and Dabco and is used to dissolve these materials to a homogeneous solution that can be efficiently and uniformly mixed with the resin. Because it dissolves the two components at room temperature, it is not necessary to use high temperatures to liquefy the TMP and the Dabco catalyst.

- Component master batch.
- Part A — Cyanaprene A-8 resin, 300 grams.
- Part B — Trimethylopropane, 100 grams.
-       Triethylene diamine, 0.210 grams.
-       Dimethoxytetra ethylene glycol, 135 grams.
- Preheat mold at 95°C for a minimum of 60 min to ensure proper temperature stability
- Heat Part A for at least 45 min.
- Evacuate Part A for at least 45 min.
- Remove from the vacuum system and place in an oven for at least 8 min at 110°C.
- Preheat required amount of Part B to 60°C until is completely clear.
- Mix Parts A and B and stir vigorously with a mechanical mixer for 60 sec.
- Evacuate until the mixture is stable at 30 microns; not to exceed 6 mins.
- Inject into the preheated mold with dry nitrogen and precure at 110°C for 3 hr.
- Demold when cooled, and prepare for flocking. Two additional cycles of 14 hr at 110°C will be required.

The formulated urethane is a soft, flexible, rubber-like material that has excellent abrasion resistance and good flex life. It is clear, light straw color, with a durometer of 55 shore A. It can be molded into any desired form by the low-pressure, injection molding techniques. Its main disadvantage is that it is a polyester; i.e., it is subject to hydrolytic instability.

This material has been used in vivo in over 300 calf experiments. It has demonstrated reliable performance for short durations, and sporatic performance for short durations, and sporatic performance for durations of up to 9 months. In vitro testing resulted in the same performance patterns as experienced in vivo — reliable short-term performance and sporatic long-term performance, with some bladders exceeding 60×10^6 cycles.

In summary, this material exhibits the following characteristics:

Advantages

- It is resistant to abrasion.
- It can be sterilized in steam (270°F, 3 min).
- It is easily castable.
- It has been approved for short-term clinical trials [6,7].
- It is easily flocked.
- It is elastomeric.
- It is formulated under strict quality control for medical-grade application.
- It has a tensile strength of 2500 psi at 600 percent elongation.

Disadvantages

- It shows hydrolytic instability.
- It has a limited long-term flex life.
- It is permeable to water vapor.

Tecoflex HR (Thermo Electron)

To overcome the disadvantages of the Tecothane B urethane, a new family of urethane polymers was synthesized [4]. These urethanes, designated Tecoflex, are aliphatic, polyether-based, linear-segmented elastomers containing 100-percent urethane linkages in the molecular backbone. The urethane if hydrolytically stable because it is a polyether instead of a polyester. The material exhibits elastic recovery qualities because the linear urethane elastomers are rubber-like block copolymers containing relatively short, hard, crystalline segments evenly dispersed among long and flexible amorphous segments.

Tecoflex HR is a two-component polymer consisting of Hylene W, Polymeg 2000, butanediol, and dibutyl tin dilaurate. It is moldable both by two-component casting and by lacquer dipping. The first method requires no solvents since the components of the polymer have an initial low viscosity that allows for easy injection into the mold. The second method, lacquer dipping, requires that the polymer be completely synthesized and later dissolved in an appropriate solvent such as dimethyl acetamide (DMA).

The procedure used to formulate the synthesized polymer is as follows:

- Components
  Part A — Hylene W
  Part B —/Polymeg 2000
       Butanediol
       Dibutyl Tin Dilaurate
- Preheat Parts A and B to 38°C.
  Hylene W is liquid at room temperature. Polymeg 2000 is solid at room temperature and must be brought up to 38°C so that the butanediol remains in solution.
- Preheat mold to 50° to 55°C.
- Mechanically stir the solution for 2 min and dearate for 6 min.
- Before injection, allow to exotherm to 41° to 43°C.
- Keep mold at 53°C when injecting Tecoflex, and then place it in the oven for 1 hr at 55°C.
- Final cure at 110°C for 3 hr.
- Let mold cool to 50° to 60°C before extraction.

Once this procedure is completed, the Tecoflex HR can either be used as it is, or it can be further dissolved in DMA to produce a lacquer for future dipping operations.

The formulated material is clear and exhibits a strength of 4900 psi at 900-percent elongation [4]. It has a durometer of 75 shore A. Tecoflex HR has been used in vivo in over 50 calf experiments, but, because it is in such a new stage of development, the results have been inconsistent. The material will, therefore, require additional time to optimize its mechanical and biological properties.

In summary, Tecoflex HR exhibits the following characteristics:

Advantages

- It is easily castable.
- It requires no solvent.
- It is biocompatible.
- It is elastomeric.
- It is formulated under strict quality control for medical-grade application.
- It has a potential long-term flex life greater than 80×10^6 cycles.
- It can be fabricated by two techniques — lacquer dipping and two-component casting.
- It is hydrolytically stable.
- It is easily flocked.

Disadvantages
- It should not be steam sterilized.
- It has poor abrasion resistance.
- It has an inconsistent flex life.
- It is permeable to water vapor.

Two-Component Reactive Casting

This technique is utilized to fabricate components from reactive urethane polymers. Urethanes such as Tecothane or Tecoflex can easily be used with this casting procedure to fabricate reproducible and complex components. The procedure consists of preparing the prepolymer and curative, mixing, and finally injecting into a specially designed mold. The polymer is cured initially in the mold, and then post-cured after extraction.

One of the most important considerations in this molding technique is proper mold design. The mold should be fabricated from aluminum to permit uniform heat distribution and rapid temperature-cycling time. Temperature-sensing probes are incorporated directly into the mold to track mold temperatures precisely throughout the cycle. Temperature must be maintained to within 5°C for reproducible components.

Another important consideration in the mold design is that it must not have horizontal parting lines. These surface discontinuities tend to capture air bubbles, which result in voids in the finished component. Vertical parting lines are acceptable if they are precise and properly contoured. There must never be spaces where air can be trapped, and all surfaces must be angulated to allow for the free movement of air and urethane. Sharp corners, internal or external, must be avoided.

All of the urethane contact surfaces should be prepared with a Teflon-sprayed coating such as 8-403 TFE (Precision Coating). This coating provides the releasing properties necessary for removal of the cured urethane component. Because urethane tends to adhere well to uncoated metallic surfaces, the components could be damaged during the extraction phase if such a coating were not used. Molds should also be designed to incorporate sufficient excess urethane material for destructive quality control testing. With this technique, the quality of the component can be verified by evaluating the material that was fabricated under the exact same conditions as those used to fabricate the component.

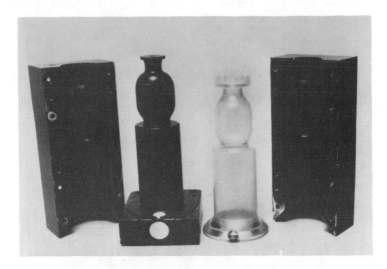

Figure 6. Typical Teflon-coated aluminum mold.

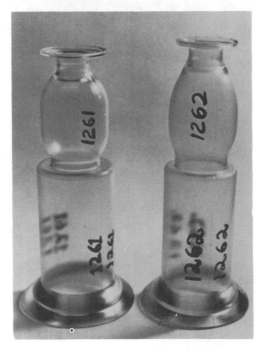

Figure 7. Urethane bladders as demolded with integral quality control material.

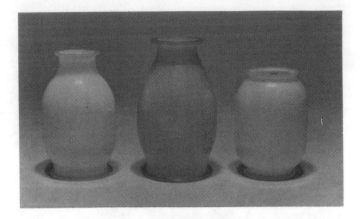

Figure 8. Completed bladders fabricated by two-component casting techniques.

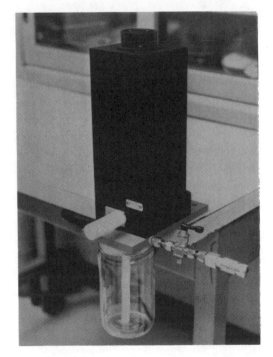

Figure 9. Closed mold positioned on filling apparatus.

Figure 6 illustrates a typical, Teflon-coated aluminum mold used for the fabrication of blood pump bladders; Figure 7 illustrates the urethane bladder with the quality control material. The bottom portion is used to destructively test the urethane to ensure that the component has been properly processed. The finished bladders, after being trimmed, are shown in Figure 8.

The next important consideration in the two-component reactive casting system is the mold-filling apparatus. As shown in Figure 9, the mold is positioned on top of the filling apparatus. The prepolymer and curative are prepared, mixed, and deaerated in a jar. The jar is attached to the filling apparatus, as shown. Dry nitrogen gas is then injected into the jar to pressurize the polymer. Approximately 3 to 5 psi is required. The pressurized polymer is then forced up through the center Teflon tube where it receives a final filtering (35 μm filter). It then enters into the base of the mold, past a one-way ball valve, and into the mold cavity. The polymer continues to fill the mold until it enters a reservoir cavity mounted on the uppermost part of the mold. At this time, the pressure is released from the jar and filling ceases. The urethane is held in the mold because of the one-way ball valve positioned at the mold base. The filled mold is then transported to an air-circulating oven for curing.

Proper preparation of the prepolymer and curative system is crucial to the successful fabrication of reliable urethane components. The prepolymer is heated initially in an air-circulating oven to liquefy. It is then carefully filtered, separated to the proper batch size, aerated in a vacuum system, and reheated in an oven to maintain the proper temperature. The curative system is likewise filtered, prepared in the proper batch size, and heated to the proper temperature. The next step in the cycle consists of mixing the prepolymer and the curative system. Severe mixing is required to disperse the curative uniformly into the prepolymer.

After mixing, the polymer is again deaerated in a vacuum system until all of the air is released. The temperature is carefully monitored and maintained at the proper level by heating or cooling, as required. At the proper point in the cycle, the container is attached to the filling apparatus and the polymer is injected into the preheated mold cavity. The mold is then transferred to an air-circulating oven and maintained at temperature for a length of time sufficient to cure the polymer. At this point, the component is demolded and subsequently post-cured to complete the polymerization.

Throughout the molding cycle, it is imperative that cleanliness be maintained at the highest level to prevent inclusions of foreign particles. The molding facility should be under positive pressure and equipped with deep-bed filters to prevent airborne particles from entering the facility. Only filtered air entering through the deep-bed filters is permitted. In addition, the humidity level of the air should be maintained between 40 and 50 percent. High humidity can cause the formation of undesirable urea bonds in the urethane.

Quality control procedures must be maintained throughout the fabrication cycle. In-process testing and evaluation must be factored into the process cycle. Temperature, humidity, and time must be closely controlled or maintained. Testing for color and viscosity of the prepolymer and curative system is done routinely, as is testing of the polymerized urethane. Microtensile test specimens are used to destructively test the urethane throughout the cycle. Tensile strength and elongation, as well as hardness, are used to ensure maintenance of the proper cycle during processing. Deviations in the cycle or material show up as variations in these parameters. Figure 10 illustrates a typical quality control procedure for the fabrication of flocked Tecothane bladders. Specific procedures must be established for every material because the requirements vary from material to material.

Biomer (Ethicon)

Biomer is a segmented polyether polyurethane polymer offered as 30 percent solution in DMA. It is known to be an elastomer possessing excellent strength and flex-life endurance. Biomer films are essentially inert in living tissue and relatively nonthrombogenic in the vascular system.

Although the exact composition of Biomer remains proprietary to its producer, it is believed that the soft segment of the molecule is based on poly tetra methylene ether glycol and that the hard segments are composed of a mixture of methylene di isocyanate (MDI) and a diamine coupler [5].

This urethane can be used only with lacquer dipping techniques. It is a clear, straw-colored elastomer with a strength of 6000 psi at 800-percent elongation. The durometer of the material is 75 shore A. The material has been in use for over 10 years and has proven to be a superior biomedical elastomer. Flex data accumulated thus far for fabricated bladders has exceeded 320×10^6 cycles [8]. When properly fabricated, it is a reliable material.

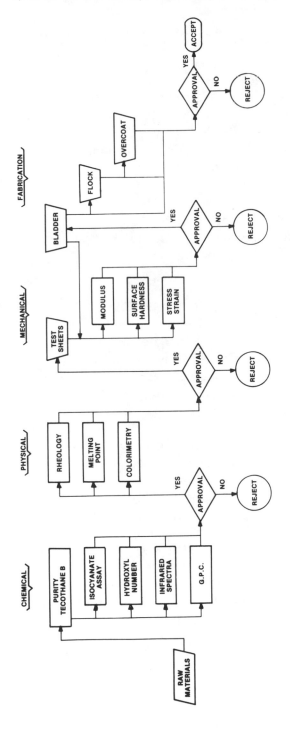

Figure 10. Simplified quality assurance procedures for flocked tecothane bladders.

In summary, this material exhibits the following characteristics:

Advantages
- It can be sterilized in steam.
- It is biocompatible.
- It is reliable.
- It is elastomeric.
- It has an excellent flex life, greater than 320×10^6 cycles.
- It is suitable for medical-grade application.
- It exhibits hydrolytic stability.
- It is easily flocked.

Disadvantages
- It is permeable to water vapor.
- It is difficult to fabricate reproducible complex parts.
- It shows poor abrasion resistance.

LACQUER DIPPING

One class of urethanes are formulated as pure lacquers; i.e., they are available only as fully cured polymers dissolved in an appropriate solvent. These materials cannot be cast in molds because they undergo too great a volume change as the solvent is removed. One such material is Biomer (Ethicon). This material is available only as a solution containing 30 percent Biomer in DMA. For proper utilization of the material, the components must be designed in a geometry that will allow for the immersion of a mandrel into the dissolved Biomer. Multiple immersions result in a film that represents the desired shape.

Three variations of the dipping technique can be utilized. The first technique, vertical dipping, consists of slowly immersing a mandrel into the solution of Biomer to obtain a desired film. The mandrel must be shaped to prevent excessive axial flow; otherwise, the urethane will flow down and accumulate at the bottom of the mandrel, resulting in varying film thicknesses from top to bottom. To overcome this problem, the mandrel can be inverted after each dip. When mandrel geometries are nonuniform in the radial direction (i.e., when they are square or noncylindrical in shape), then they must be dipped in a vertical direction to avoid nonuniform film thicknesses. Figure 11 illustrates a typical mandrel in the process of being immersed.

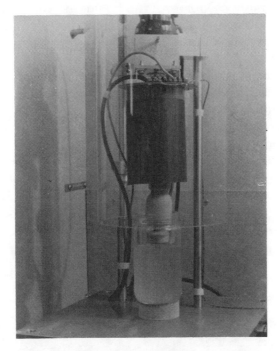

Figure 11. Mandrel being immersed into biomer lacquer.

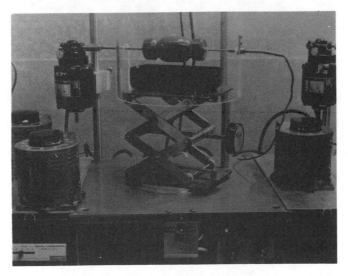

Figure 12. Horizontal dipping into biomer lacquer.

The second method of dipping can be utilized with mandrels that are not consistent in the axial direction but that are cylindrical in the radial direction. The technique consists of rotating the mandrel in a horizontal position while slowly immersing it into the Biomer solution. After two complete rotations, the mandrel is slowly removed and the film is allowed to dry. This, again, produces a film of uniform thickness. Figure 12 illustrates this technique.

The third technique is used to fabricate planner diaphragms or sheets. It consits of mounting a disc of the appropriate shape to the head stock of a standard lathe. A contoured doctor blade, mounted to the compound is then brought to within 0.2 mm of the disc while Biomer is being applied with a syringe. The disc is rotated while the doctor blade is slowly retracted and all of the Biomer is attached to the disc. Nonuniform thicknesses can be obtained with this technique simply by adjusting the spacing and contour of the doctor blade. Figure 13 illustrates this technique.

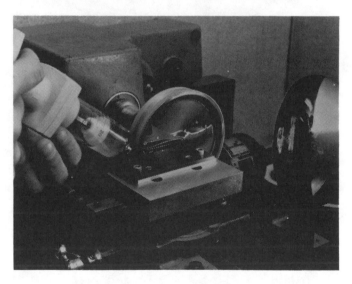

Figure 13. Template-formed biomer diaphragms.

The mandrels or disc should be fabricated from aluminum and coated with a release agent. Either TFE or mold release agents are effective. The actual fabrication should be conducted in a hooded area for the proper removal of DMA. Figure 14 illustrates a typical facility in which all three techniques can be accomplished.

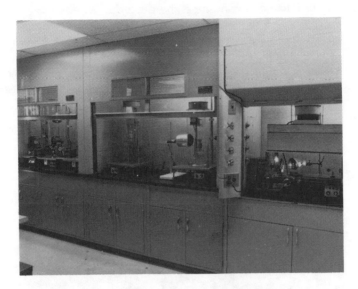

Figure 14. Biomer dipping facility.

Cleanliness is again a major factor. The fabrication stations are arranged in such a way that only filtered air is used during the dipping stages. Heat lamps are used to control temperatures, and dipping and filtered-air circulating ovens are utilized for the drying phases.

Biomer is a true lacquer. It is obtained from the manufacturer as a 30-percent solution of Biomer in DMA. For processing, the polymer is further reduced by adding DMA until a viscosity of 1500 centipoises at 50°C is obtained. At this point, the Biomer is filtered through a 30-μm filter while being transferred to the working containers. These loaded containers are maintained at 50°C for the remainder of the cycle.

The aluminum mandrel is maintained at a temperature just slightly less than 50°C. It is then slowly immersed (1.7 cm/min) into the Biomer until the mandrel is completely coated. It is then slowly extracted (1.7 cm/min) and placed in an oven to remove the solvents. This drying time is between 60 and 90 min. The resulting film thickness, after drying, should be approximately 0.07 mm. This dipping and drying cycle is continued until the desired thickness is obtained. At this point, the bladder is removed from the mandrel and dried for an additional 5 hr at 50°C.

One of the major difficulties encountered with this material is in the fabrication of components with nonuniform thickness. To overcome this problem, the bladder must be fabricated in two steps. To fabricate a bladder with a thick flange, for instance, the procedure consists of first manufacturing a sheet of Biomer by the template-forming procedure. Next, the sheet is machined to the appropriate geometry (ring), and the finished component is mounted onto the dipping mandrel. The ring must be machined slightly smaller than the mandrel in order to be in tension on the mandrel. If the ring is not in tension, rapid swelling during immersion results in movement and excessive solvation. The mandrel, with rings positioned, is then dipped in the usual manner. When the ring contacts the DMA solvent, surface solvation occurs and results in a chemical bond to the Biomer solution. A typical flange formed by this procedure is shown in Figure 15.

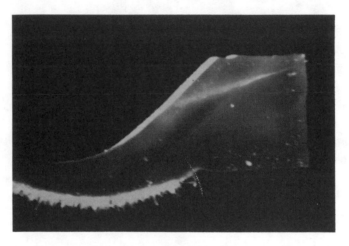

Figure 15. Flange biomer-formed by a two-step process.

TEXTURED SURFACE

Introduction

Numerous materials have been considered for use as blood-interaction surfaces in prosthetic devices. These have been classified in five broad categories: (1) synthetic materials, such as ionic, polarized, or neutral polymers and pyrolytic carbons; (2) synthetic materials with additives, such as heparin and surface active agents; (3) hydrogels, both neutral and anionic; (4) textured surfaces, such as flock, velour, and microfiber scaffold, which initiate a substrate for neointima development; and (5) composites based on combinations of the above. Thermo Electron's work in the area of blood-compatible surfaces, being carried out in conjunction with the development of left ventricular assist pumps, has concentrated on the textured-surface approach.

In our early work (1968) with assist pumps, the flexible bladders were fabricated from smooth, molded silicone rubber with no surface treatment. Five animal pump experiments were conducted with this type of surface [9]; within 3 to 5 days, the surface was covered with a progressively thickening layer of thrombus (despite anticoagulation), and extensive systemic embolization was observed. Additionally, there was evidence of gross hemolysis throughout each study. These discouraging results prompted investigations of surfaces that promote formation of a biologic interface.

The previous efforts of Liotta, DeBakey, and coworkers [10, 11, 12], who utilized Dacron velour cloth to promote the growth of an organized fibrin layer, provided a basis for our initial work. Although satisfactory short-term results were obtained with the Dacron velour, thrombus accumulation and scattered areas of calcification were observed. In our evaluation, these problems were related to the thick pile depth of the velour.

Our approch to the problem consisted of lining the internal blood-contacting surfaces of the pump with short polyester fibrils to promote the adhesion of a thick fibrinous coagulum. The original work was carried out with fibrils 500 μm long, but, later (and up to the present time), fibrils 300 μm in length were used, with improved results. Polyester fibrils applied in a random manner are attached to the substrate (either metal or elastomer) by means of a cross-linked polyurethane adhesive. Some initial problems were encountered with long-term adherence of the flock matrix to the flexing substrates; however, the techniques currently employed give a high degree of reliability for several months' operation, and successful implants in excess of 9 months' duration have been achieved.

Over 500 studies have been carried out using flocked surfaces of this type in claves with assist devices. The neointima that formed on a flock-matrix of 500-μm fibrils has been consistently thicker than that formed on a matrix of 300-μm fibrils. This observation is in agreement with that of other workers [13] and suggests that optimum fiber size may be smaller than that currently being used.

Although the precise mechanism of pseudointima formation is not totally understood, a large body of knowledge has been accumulated over the years, which allows some explanation of kinetic events. There is general agreement that certain plasma proteins coat the surface of any substance exposed to blood. This conditioning monomolecular layer is deposited within seconds, and greatly influences subsequent occurrences.

The plasma proteins that adsorb on the surface of polyurethanes are gamma globulins, fibrinogen, and albumin. In some cases, where albumin is preferentially adsorbed, the surface undergoes a passivation process, remaining in a state of dynamic equilibrium. In other cases, where fibrinogen is adsorbed, it undergoes polymerization to fibrin, attracting platelets, which leads to thrombus formation. Adsorption of plasma proteins into polymeric surfaces is currently an area of intense scientific investigation.

When a flocked surface is exposed to blood, there is little doubt that plasma proteins are adsorbed onto each polyester fibril. Within several minutes, platelets adhere and agglomerate in the interstices of the flocked matrix. Shortly thereafter, a sticky network of fibrin is deposited between the platelets, attracting and retaining circulating erythrocytes and leukocytes. This process continues until all the exposed fibrins are covered, and the lining then ceases to grow.

This initial thrombus is capable of flexing, and, since it was derived from the blood itself, it is nonthrombogenic. After 2 or 3 months, fibroblasts penetrate the lining, colonize, and begin to synthesize collagen. With the passage of time, collagen slowly replaces fibrin, resulting in a stable pseudoendothelial lining.

Random Flocking Techniques

Flocking techniques were established to form stable textured blood-interaction surfaces. Commercially available flock, 300 μm by 17 μm, is available in polyester, such as polyethylene terephthalate (Dacron) material. This flock is coated with a proprietary coating to achieve free-flowing properties, which is required for proper application. This coating must be removed before the material can be used on a blood pump. In any implantable device, care must be taken to use only nontoxic materials whose reproducibility can be completely controlled.

The finish is stripped from the flock by vigorous stirring in a solution of

Acationox, sodium carbonate, and distilled water. The solution is heated to 100°C and the pH maintained at 10. Multiple washes are required, with final rinsing in distilled water. The cleaned flock is then collected in a Whatman No. 31 low-ash filter paper. Stripped flock is then examined with a scanning electron microscope (SEM) at 1000x to ensure that the finish has been completely removed.

The stripped flock is then recoated with another finish, which is prepared under controlled conditions. Twenty liters of dionized water is brought up to a temperature of 50°C. One-hundred grams of Leomin KP Type F (American Hoechst) is added with 400 grams of anhydrous sodium sulfate and 30 grams of aluminum potassium sulfate.

One thousand grams of stripped flock is then added to the solution and stirred. Sodium carbonate is added to achieve a pH of 8 to 8.5, and stirring continues for 25 to 30 min. The flock is then filtered and dried for 14 hr at 65°C. The dried flock is separated, by passing it through a 28-mesh filter, and stored.

The flock is then inspected under SEM at 1000x to determine the amount of finish added. The finish will appear as droplets on the fiber. In addition, the weight of finish "add-on" is determined. About 5 grams of flock is placed in a dried and weighed extraction thimble. The weight is documented to four decimals. The finish is then extracted for 4 hr with boiling, deionized water in a Soxhlet extraction apparatus. The thimble is dried at 100°C for 2 hr and weighed; the percentage of weight loss is calculated and recorded. The extract is evaporated to dryness in a rotary evaporator, and the recovered material is calculated as a percentage of the dry fiber.

The specific flocking technique is dependent on the type of base material; the adhesive that is used must be designed for the particular application. Different adhesives are used for Biomer, Tecothane, and Tecoflex HR substrates. Curing durations and temperatures are also adjusted to meet the particular requirements of the adhesive being used.

As an example, the flocking procedure for Biomer bladders is as follows:

- Mount the bladder in an appropriate Teflon-coated fixture, leaving exposed only those surfaces to be coated.
- Prepare Biomer flocking adhesive A-457-13 (Thermo Electron) by carefully weighing 100 parts of prepolymer to 50 parts of chain extender. The mixed compound has a nominal working life of 2 hr.
- Spray exposed surfaces of the bladder, finger uniformly, and let stand for approximately 10 min.

- After the flocking adhesive has flowed uniformly over the surface of the bladder, spray once again lightly and dust flock fibers on immediately.
- Let the bladder stand at room temperature for approximately 10 min and dust once again before placing in the oven for 5 hr at 110°C.

After curing, the bladder must be processed further to remove any loose fibrils and all of the finish used previously. The finish that was applied to the fibers was necessary to prevent agglomeration; however, once the fibers have been adhesively bonded, it is no longer necessary and should be removed because it is water soluble.

To remove the loose fibrils and flock finish, the bladder is immersed in one quart of 20-percent isopropyl alcohol and deionized water, and is sonicated for 30 min. The supernatant liquid, with free fibrils and other impurities, is discarded. The bladder is then rinsed thoroughly with deionized water and again placed in one quart of fresh deionized water and sonicated for 30 min. The supernatant fluid should be absent of fibrils or other debris. The bladder is then placed in a circulating oven and dried for 30 min at 110°C. Examination of the stripped bladder under SEM should yield a bladder appearance as shown in Figures 16 and 17. Voids at the adhesive fiber interface should be present; since the adhesive was bonded to the finish and not the fibril, removal of the finish, of course, leaves voids, which will subsequently be filled with an overcoat varnish.

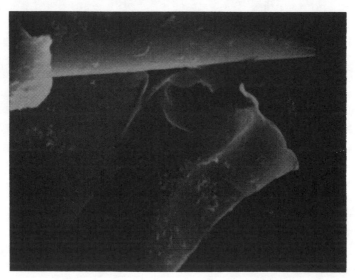

Figure 16. Fiber-to-adhesive bonds after washing and prior to overcoating (2000×).

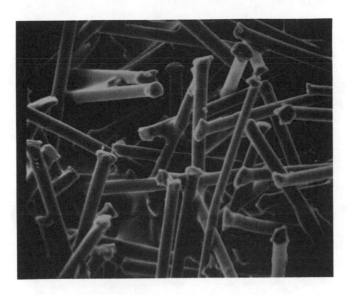

Figure 17.   Fiber-to-adhesive bonds after washing and prior to overcoating (200×).

The next procedure in the cycle consists of overcoating [14] the flock matrix with a diluted solution of urethane adhesive. The varnish (A-457-14 Thermo Electron) is prepared by mixing 100 parts by weight of the prepolymer and 100 parts by weight of chain extender. The mixed compound should be used within 2 hr to avoid gelation. The varnish is put into a syringe and applied to the fibrils. As the varnish wets the flock matrix, a distinct color change occurs. This color change is used as a guide to ensure that all of the fibrils are saturated with the overcoat solution. The bladder is then cured for 6 hr at 110°C in a vacuum desiccator.

The surface of the finished bladder, inspected under SEM, should be similar in appearance to those shown in Figures 18 and 19. As can be seen, all of the voids have been filled and the fibrils rebonded to the substrate. In addition, secondary bonds have been formed at all contact points between fibrils. The overall appearance of the flock surface should be as shown in Figure 20.

The bladder is then ready for final cleaning. It is immersed in distilled water and sonicated for 30 min. The fluid is discarded and fresh distilled water added. The bladder is sonicated for an additional 30 min. At this point, there should be no fibrils or particulate residue in the water. Examination under intense light should reveal a clear fluid with no foreign particles. The bladder is then dried and packaged in a polyethylene bag.

Victor Poirier

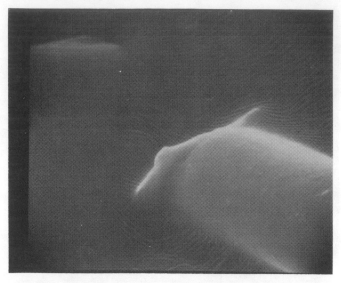

Figure 18. Fiber-to-adhesive bonds after overcoating with dilute solution of polyurethane (2000 ×).

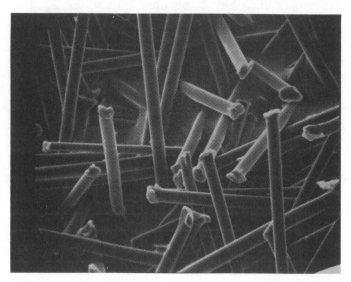

Figure 19. Fiber-to-adhesive bonds after overcoating with dilute solution of polyurethane (200 ×).

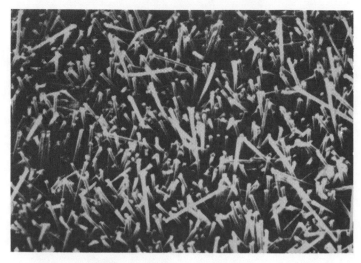

Figure 20. SEM photograph of manually flocked surface (50 ×).

Integral Flock Techniques

An improvement to the random flocking of polyester fibrils is the integral flock technique. The technique consists of forming the flock fibrils as an integral part of the base substrate. In essence, the flock fibrils and the base substrate are of the same material and are continuous in nature. No adhesives or finish are used.

Integral-flock Biomer bladders [15] are fabricated according to the method shown diagrammatically in Figure 21. The process consists of producing a transfer mold of Silastic J (Dow Corning) which has been cast against an electrostatically flocked master mandrel. The inner surface of the master mold if flocked with nylon monofilaments, 3 denier in diameter, precision cut to 300 μm in length.

After electrostatic flocking, the Silastic J mixture is poured into the master mandrel and allowed to cure at room temperature for 24 hr. After curing, the silicone transfer mold is separated from the master mandrel, as shown in Figure 22. At this stage, the nylon monofilaments are embedded into the silicone transfer mold. The transfer mold is placed into a 30-percent solution of phenol/methylene chloride, which preferentially dissolves the embedded monofilaments but is innocuous to the silicone. A negative-replica silicone mold is obtained once all the monofilaments

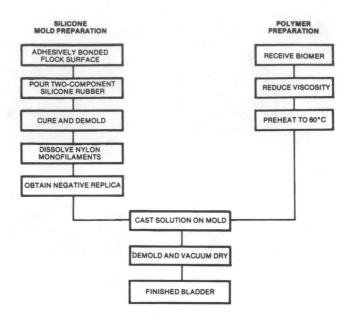

Figure 21. Diagrammatic representation depicting steps in manufacture of integrally textured surfaces.

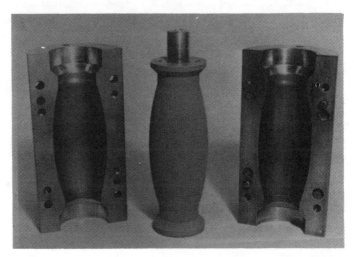

Figure 22. Silicone rubber transfer mandrel flanked by open halves of the master mold.

have been dissolved, leaving a surface replete with invaginations, which represent the volume once occupied by the monofilaments. A close-up view of silicone transfer mold is shown in Figure 23.

Integrally textured (IT) bladders are fabricated by successively immersing the negative-replica silicone transfer mold into a low-viscosity Biomer solution. The apparatus used for this purpose is shown in Figure 24. The facilities utilized for Biomer bladder fabrication are depicted in Figure 14. By this method, a high-fidelity facsimile of conventionally flocked surfaces is obtained, as seen in Figure 25; for comparison purposes, a conventionally flocked surface is shown in Figure 26.

Alternate Matrix Thickness

Development work was carried out to produce alternate matrix thicknesses to arrive at an optimal configuration. The first matrix thickness that was developed was 430 μm thick. This surface was used to evaluate the IT surface against the standard polyester-flocked surfaces. Results were encouraging in that the biologically formed linings were consistent and uniform.

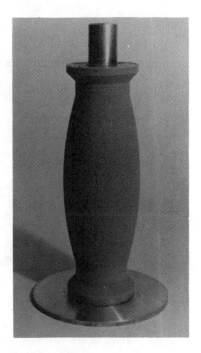

Figure 23. Close-up view of bladder-shaped transfer mandrel.

Two additional matrix thicknesses were developed, as shown in Table 2. These surfaces are progressively thinner and produce thinner biologic lining. The first matrix, although quite thick, has proven to be satisfactory, which suggests that cells are nourished not only by diffusion through the lining but also by mass transport through the pseudointima. Thinner linings are advantageous to assure cellular viability and reduce mechanical stress levels. The thinner the lining, the lower the membrane stresses that are produced during constant flexure.

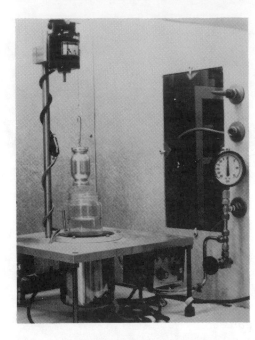

Figure 24. Vertical sequential casting of biomer bladders.

Table 2. Dimensional and Functional Characteristics of Integrally Textured Biomer Bladders Model 11S

0.030" Starting Monofilament

- Fibril dimensions   0.018 mm diameter x 0.51 mm length
- Fibril density   135 fibrils/mm^2
- Internal wetted surface area with fibril 5.318×10^4 mm^2
- Mat thickness   0.43 mm

0.020" Starting Monofilament

- Fibril dimensions   0.018 mm diameter x 0.38 mm length
- Fibril density   135 fibrils/mm^2
- Internal wetted surface area with fibril 4.262×10^4 mm^2
- Mat thickness   0.31 mm

0.010" Starting Monofilament

- Fibril dimensions   0.018 mm diameter x 0.23 mm length
- Fibril density   220 fibrils/mm^2
- Internal wetted surface area with fibril 3.835×10^4 mm^2
- Mat thickness   0.20 mm

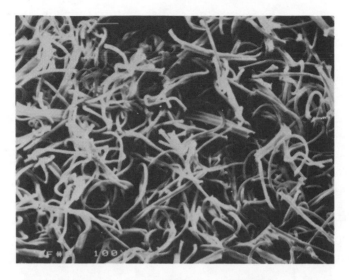

Figure 25. Integrally textured biomer surface obtained by dip casting (100×).

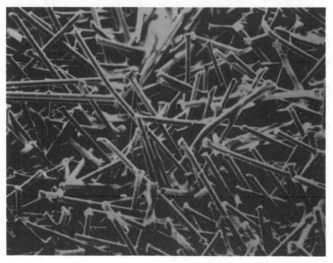

Figure 26. Conventionally flocked surface (×100).

ENDURANCE TESTING OF TEXTURED BLADDERS

One of the major criteria of any blood-pump bladder is that it must withstand flexure at the rate of 40×10^6 cycles per year. To evaluate bladders for this requirement, they must undergo real-time endurance testing in a manner that replicates, as closely as possible, the actual in vivo use.

Methods

To evaluate bladders, a comprehensive endurance test was undertaken. The evaluation factored not only the materials but the effects of geometrical shape. Seven materials, shown in Figure 27, and eight geometries, shown in Figure 28, were evaluated in test loops [16], as illustrated in Figures 29 and 30. The pumps were operated at beat rates between 80 and 160 beats per min, pumping saline at 39°C into a pressure head of 100 mm Hg. The pumps were operated at full-design stroke volumes ranging from 75 to 85 ml, depending on the particular model being tested.

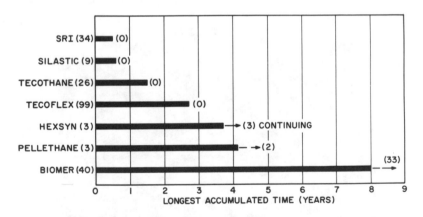

Figure 27. Longest accumulated time of the seven test materials.

The materials that were evaluated consisted of the following: 1) 34 bladders of SRI 3-20001 — this material is a linear segmented, ether-type urethane supplied in a lacquer form and manufactured by Stanford Research Institute; 2) 9 diaphragms of Silastic MDX 4-4515 — this material is a silicone rubber compound supplied in an unvulcanized state by Dow Corning; 3) 26 bladders of Tecothane B — this material is a two-component, polyester, cross-linked urethane of the cyanaprene family (American Cyanamid); it is modified and manufactured by Thermo Elec-

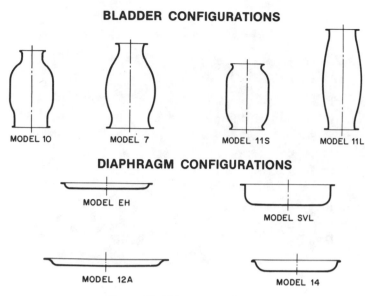

Figure 28. Eight test configurations.

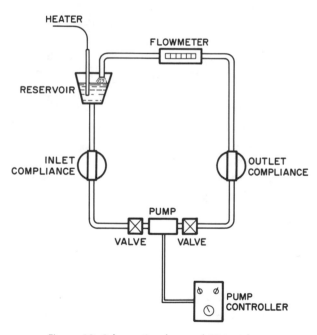

Figure 29. Schematic of one of 50 test loops.

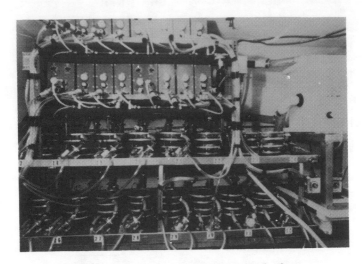

Figure 30. 16-Station endurance test facility.

tron Corporation; 4) 99 bladders and diaphragms of Tecoflex HR — this material is an aliphatic, polyether-based, linear-segmented elastomer containing 100-percent urethane linkages; it is manufactured by Thermo Electron Corporation; 5) 3 diaphragms of Hexsyn — this material is a polyolefin rubber manufactured by Goodyear Rubber; 6) 3 diaphragms of Pellethane — this material is a thermoplastic polymer whose exact composition is proprietary to Upjohn Chemical; it is supplied in pellet or sheet form and is believed to be composed of PTMEG 1,4-butanediol and MDI; 7) 40 bladders and diaphragms of Biomer — this material is a segmented polyether urethane offered as 30-percent by weight solution in DMA; although the exact composition remains proprietary by Ethicon, Inc., it is believed that the soft segments of the molecule are based on PTMEG, and that the hard segments are composed of a mixture of MDI and a diamine coupler.

RESULTS

Seven materials and eight configurations, as shown in Figure 31, were evaluated. Of these materials, Tecothane B, Tecoflex HR, Silastic, and SRI resulted in considerable variability. Figure 32 illustrates the typical raw data obtained for one of these materials and one configuration. As can be seen, bladder life varied from 1.5×10^6 cycles to 67×10^6 cycles.

Materials were evaluated in the same pump configuration to deter-

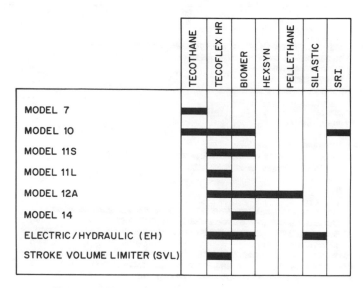

Figure 31. Materials and configuration types tested.

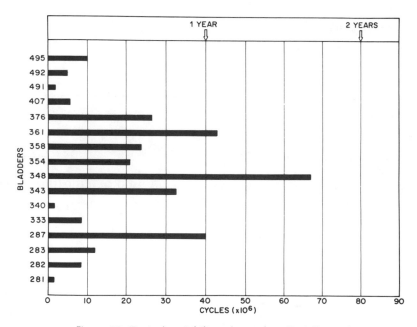

Figure 32. Typical variability of raw data (Tecoflex HR).

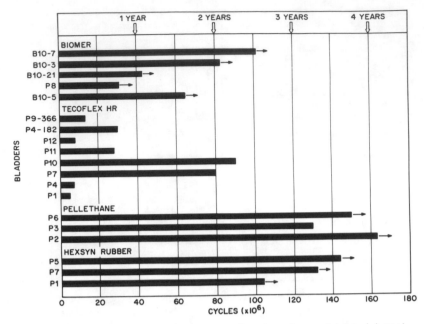

Figure 33. Assist pump endurance as a function of material (Model 12A).

mine whether material properties influence flexure endurance. Figure 33 illustrates a typical result. As expected, material properties do not affect flexure endurance.

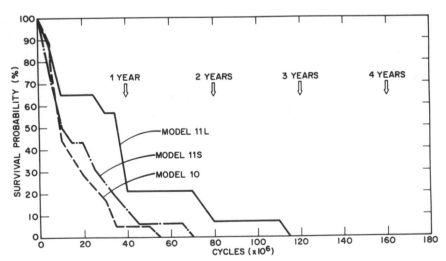

Figure 34. Effects of bladder geometry on flexure endurance (Tecoflex HR).

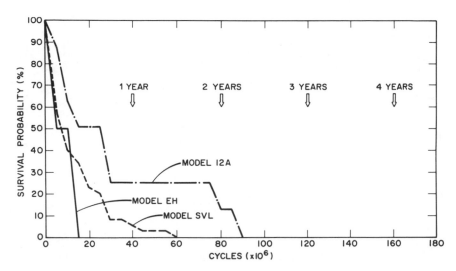

Figure 35. Effects of diaphragm geometry on flexure endurance (Tecoflex HR).

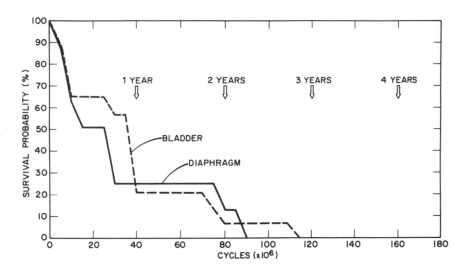

Figure 36. Comparison of the best bladder and the best diaphragm fabricated from Tecoflex HR

In conjunction, the same materials were evaluated in several geometric shapes to determine the effects of configuration. Figure 34 illustrates three different bladder geometries, and Figure 35 illustrates

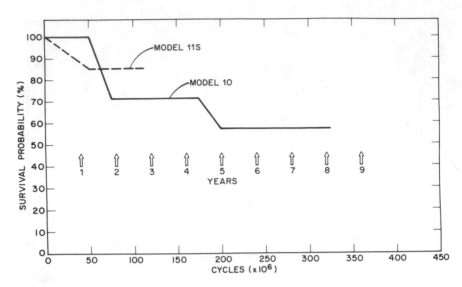

Figure 37. Comparison of bladder geometry on flexure endurance (Biomer).

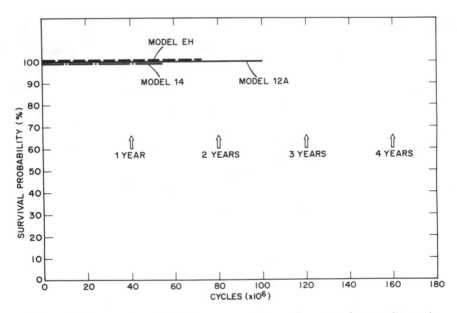

Figure 38. Comparison of diaphragm geometry on flexure endurance (Biomer).

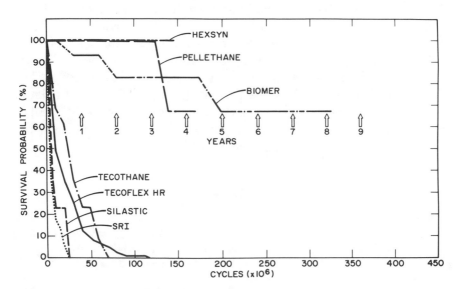

Figure 39. Flexure-endurance comparison of seven materials tested.

three different diaphragm geometries, fabricated from the same material. As expected, bladder geometry greatly affects flexure endurance. A comparison was made between the best bladder geometry and the best diaphragm geometry to determine whether geometric design could be eliminated as a parameter. Figure 36 illustrates the results. As can be seen, the two curves are quite similar (areas under curves are 8.1 versus 9.2) and indicate that, if the geometry is properly designed, the basic material property will be the deciding factor.

The most impressive materials evaluated as long-term bladders or diaphragms were Biomer, Hexsyn, and Pellethane. Unlike the previously mentioned materials, these materials gave consistent results. Two Biomer bladder geometries and three diaphragm geometries were evaluated, with the results illustrated in Figures 37 and 38. As can be seen, geometry is again a factor. No failures have been experienced with the diaphragm geometries, whereas several failures were observed with the bladder geometries. Although these failures were not basic material failures, such as material degradation or cracking, they were failures nonetheless. The bladders that failed had rubbed against the pump housing and worn through. The Biomer material is not abrasion resistant and will fail if allowed to rub against the pump housing.

To determine how one material ranked with another in terms of flexure endurance, all of the test configurations were combined and plotted against cycle life [17]. Figure 39 illustrates the results of 214 individual tests. As can be seen, two distinct groups were formed. Hexsyn, Pellethane, and Biomer were significantly superior to Tecoflex HR, Tecothane B, Silastic, and SRI. Only three diaphragms of each of the latter two types were evaluated. Considerably more data must be accumulated with these two material types before they can be considered for actual use in cardiac assist systems.

REFERENCES

1. "Dow Corning's Clean-Grade Elastomers" Bulletin No. 51-209, Medical Products Business, Dow Corning Corporation, Midland, Michigan 48640 (August 1973).
2. Poirier, V., Gernes, D., and Szycher, M., "Advances in Electrical Assist Devices," Trans. ASAIO 23:73-79 (April 1977).
3. Williams, D.F. and Roaf, R., *Implants in Surgery,* W.B. Saunders Co., London, pp. 190, 229-232, 261, 263 (1973).
4. Szycher, M., Poirier, V., and Keiser, J., "Selection of Materials for Ventricular Assist Pump Development and Fabrication," Trans. ASAIO, 23:116-126 (April 1977).
5. Lyman, D.J., Brash, J.L., and Klein, K.G., "The Effect of Chemical Structure and Surface Properties of Synthetic Polymers on the Coagulation of Blood," in Proc. of Artif. Heart Prog. Conf., NIH, Washington, D.C., pp. 113-119 (1969).
6. Bernhard, W.F., Poirier, V., LaFarge, C.G., and Carr, J.G., "A New Method for Temporary Left Ventricular Bypass: Preclinical Appraisal," J. Thorac. Cardiovasc. Surg., 70(5):880-895 (November 1975).
7. Poirier, V.L. and Bernhard, W.F., "A Clinical Left Ventricular Assist Device," Proc. Eng. in Med. and Biology, 28:354 (September 1975).
8. Poirier, V., Szycher, M., and Whalen, R., "Comprehensive, Real Time, Endurance Testing of Cardiac Assist Pump Bladders," Trans. ASAIO (1979: in press).
9. Bernhard, W.F., et al., Annals of Surgery, 168:750 (1968).
10. DeBakey, M.E., Liotta, D., and Hall, C.W., *Mechanical Devices to Assist the Failing Heart,* National Academy of Sciences National Research Council, Washington, DC, (1966).
11. Liotta, D., et al., Cardiovascular Res. Bulletin, 4:69 (1966).
12. Hall, C.W., et al., J. Biomedical Material Research, 1:179 (1967).
13. Sharp, W.V., et al., Trans. ASAIO, 18:232 (1972).
14. Poirier, V. and Keiser, J., "Artificial Implant with Fiber-Flocked Blood-Contacting Surface," Patent No. 4,084,255 (April 18, 1978).
15. Szycher, M., Bernhard, W.F., Liss, R., and Keiser, J.T., *Development and Testing of Flocking Materials,* Annual Progress Report No. NO1-HV-2915-4, Thermo Electron Corporation, Waltham, MA (April 1977).

16. Keiser, J. and Poirier, V., *Fabrication of Implantable Artificial Heart Devices and Components*, Report No. NIH-NHLBI-71-2065-6, Thermo Electron Corporation, Waltham, MA (March 1977).
17. Association for the Advancement of Medical Instrumentation, *Pacemaker Standard: Labeling Requirements, Performance Requirements, and Terminology for Implantable Artificial Cardiac Pacemakers*, NTIS No. PB-252-607 (August 1975).

PARYLENE COATED POLYPROPYLENE MICROFIBERS AS CELL SEEDING SUBSTRATES

F.R. Tittmann
Development Scientist
and
W.F. Beach
Group Leader

Union Carbide Corporation
Chemicals & Plastics Division
One River Road
Bound Brook, New Jersey 08805
(201) 356-8000

ABSTRACT

Union Carbide, under contract with the National Heart, Lung, and Blood Institute, has developed a unique synthetic microfiber fabric for use in blood circulatory assist devices. This microfabric is at present a superior candidate material for achieving blood compatibility in cardiovascular prostheses by the neointimal tissue scaffolding approach. The fabric is a nonwoven highly porous network, approximately 25 microns thick, of polypropylene fibers about 1 micron in diameter. It is bonded to the nonporous wall of the prosthesis with an adhesive, and made suitable for the attachment and growth of tissue cells by a vapor deposited conformal coating of parylene C, followed by an electrical discharge treatment. Various animal testing and cell culture laboratories have extensively evaluated the microfabric as substrates for cultured, autologous endothelial cell linings, both in vitro and in animals as the surfaces of aortic grafts of axisymmetric blood pump bladders in left ventricular assist devices. Further characterization and development of the neointimal lining approach is under way.

This research is supported by Contract No. NO1-HV-8-1388, National Heart, Lung, and Blood Institute, Division of Heart and Vascular Diseases, Bethesda, Maryland 20014.

KEYWORDS

Microfibers, polypropylene; nonwoven fabric; ultrathin; immiscible polymer. Extrusion; lay-flat tubular film; extraction; transverse drafting; vertical drafting; tentering. Freeze-drying; parylene; vapor deposition; conformal coating. Vascular prosthesis; neointima; tissue culture; blood compatibility; endothelial cells; thrombogenicity.

INTRODUCTION

The prevention of thrombus buildup within artificial cardiovascular and circulatory assist components is a problem that is receiving intensive attention by the scientific community in the Artificial Heart Program of the National Heart, Lung, and Blood Institute (NHLBI) [1]. A technically promising route under investigation is the use of tissue culture techniques [1–14] in conjunction with an artificial surface in order to create a living cellular interface that can survive the rigors of natural cyclic pressure changes in long-term *in vivo* applications. Various artificial material surfaces have been tried for cells to grow on [1,2]. Our participation in the biomaterials phase of the program has been the approach of using a unique nonwoven fabric of ultrafine polypropylene fibers for lining the blood contacting surfaces of a nonporous prosthetic device [1,11]. The microfabric is attached by adhesive to the wall, then parylene C coated and surface treated with an electrical discharge. Appropriate cells of the host individual are subsequently grown within the fibers interstitial network and form a continuous outer blood compatible surface.

The microfiber fabric is used to meet the following biologic requirements for a satisfactory artificial implant [2,10,15,16,17]:

1) A surface should be provided to which cells readily adhere and on which they will readily grow.

2) The fabric should be sufficiently porous to allow adequate penetration of cells and fluid circulation for their survival during the *in vitro* culture period.

3) The fabric pore size should be small enough for the cells to bridge.

4) The fibers themselves should be of smaller diameter than the cells for their adherence.

5) The cellular network should be thin enough so that the innermost cells are nourished by diffusion of nutrients from the blood.

6) It is necessary to bond the fabric to suitable materials of construction for circulatory assist devices without destroying fabric porosity.

7) The fibers or fabrication components cannot exude materials toxic to cells.

BACKGROUND

This program was initiated using two novel technologies previously developed in our laboratories [2,12]:

1) A means of producing the required random network of ultrathin synthetic fibers.

2) A vapor deposited polymer, parylene, which has the unusual ability to conformally coat complex surfaces with unequaled thinness and uniformity, providing good protection as a diffusion barrier in addition to making a good network reinforcement and bond for a nonwoven fragile microfiber fabric.

The basic techniques and technical protocols for producing microfiber fabric were developed in the first phase of the program [2,12]. Cell culture studies and exploratory short-term *in vivo* tests with nonporous vascular grafts in animals indicated the parylene C coated microfiber material to have potential utility as scaffolding in the so-called neointimal lining approach to the blood compatibilization problem. From a materials standpoint, success seemed to be partly due to the mechanical properties of the polypropylene and to the parylene coating which holds the microfibers together. In particular, the living cells in direct contact with parylene surfaces exhibit no adverse effects.

The studies since then have been primarily the development of procedures to fabricate microfiber lined blood pump device components of interest to the Contract Office, and additionally the production of microfiber lined specimens for evaluation purposes. Biological assessments have entailed the fabric both *in vitro* as substrates for cultured autologous endothelial cell linings and in animals as the surfaces of implanted nonporous vascular grafts and left ventricular assist device (LVAD) bladders.

During the course of developing and producing functional microfiber lined cardiovascular devices, several problems were encountered. These related to blood compatibility, microfiber lining fabrication, and mechanical durability in repeated flexure:

1) The need to improve the microfibers surface for satisfactory adherence and growth of cells.

2) Techniques required development for applying fabric to the inner surfaces of the graft and blood pump devices.

3) Long-term attachment of fabric to the device backing in repeated flexure and stretching was unsatisfactory.

4) Physical methods were needed to predict performance of candidate microfiber linings in biological systems.

The first objective was accomplished early in the program by increasing hydrophilicity of the parylene C coated microfibers through treatment with electrical discharge, e.g. microwave glow discharge [12]. Published data have shown that wetted surfaces improve cell attachment [13]. Solutions to the remaining problems were developed. For example, a special elastomer adhesive system was formulated for use in attachment of fabrics to device backings, and also in fabrication of blood pump bladder linings [14]. It was important to achieve satisfactory bonding without the adhesive bleeding into the fiber web and engulfment thereof. Flex life testing of microfiber lined bladders in water filled mock loops, at both Thermo Electron Corporation (TECO) and our laboratories, has aided in studying mechanical integrity under repeated flexing and stretching [11,14].

MATERIALS AND METHODS

Cell Seeding Substrate Methodology

Generation of the microfibers starts with an incompatible mix of polypropylene, ethylene/acrylic acid copolymer salt (ionomer) and glycerine. The mixture is extruded and uniaxial stretched to form an oriented thin film (precursor tape). Extraction of the ionomer and glycerine, followed by transverse drafting underwater, gives a water-swollen mat of polypropylene random microfiber mesh. This is converted by freeze-drying and tentering to a nonwoven thin polypropylene microfibers web (microfabric) of gossamer nature. The final dimensions (primarily thickness and fiber network density) of unsupported fabric produced in this manner depend on the original thickness of extruded tape, degree of molecular orientation, and extent of transverse drafting. Fabrics are normally about 25 microns thick, and consist of microfibers about 1 micron thick. The fibrous network is reinforced by a very light precoat (<1500Å) of parylene C to enhance handleability. This fabric, after bonding with adhesive to the device backing, is rendered suitable for attachment and growth of tissue cells by an overcoat of parylene C followed by glow discharge treatment in Argon.

Preparation of Microfiber Fabric. Manufacture of microfiber fabric material comprises seven main steps which are described below. Complete details will be found in the references [2,11,12]:

Preparation of Immiscible Polymer Compound – Polypropylene, ionomer and glycerine are mixed by single screw compounding in the molten state to form a suspension of polypropylene droplets (approximately 10 microns diameter) in the ionomer/glycerine matrix. The mixture contains 55-60 weight percent of polypropylene.

Film Extrusion – The solidified polymer blend from the above step is single screw melt extruded and drawn as a flat film to shape the polypropylene particles into dispersed fibers aligned parallel to the extrusion direction, and embedded in the ionomer/glycerine phase. Tubular film apparatus is used for this operation. Here, the extruder is equipped with an annular die and center air mandrel. The polymer compound is extruded as a thin walled tube, and drawn while molten over the air mandrel. The tube formed is continuously collapsed by nip rolls into a tubular lay-flat laminated film.

The extrusion step, unlike the customary practice of blowing tubular polyolefin film, is designed for no diametral inflation of the tube leaving the die. In operation, the extruding tubular film is pulled longitudinally (away) from the die with minimum stretching in the transverse direction. Longitudinal stretch forms desirable thread domains of polypropylene. Should transverse stretching occur, these become lamellae and impede subsequent satisfactory extraction of the ionomer/glycerine components.

Precursor Tape Preparation – The extruded film is molecularly oriented by hot stretching it longitudinally over 900 percent to form the polypropylene threads into high tensile strength, long ultrafine fibers about 1 micron diameter, directed lengthwise along the resultant precursor tape. The process is carried out through an orientation line consisting of a radiantly heated vertical stack, and a film web handling train of controlled differential speed unwind and take-up rolls.

Wet Drafting to Form Microfiber Mesh – The ionomer and glycerine are removed from the precursor tape with hot aqueous alkali. Working in a water bath at room temperature, the extracted tape is hand drafted transversely, i.e. by pulling opposite edges apart in the direction perpendicular to the extrusion direction of the fibers. Generally, tapes are stretched at least 100-fold to obtain essentially complete randomization of the fibers. The tapes are wound onto a roll, like gauze. Drafting is carried out by repeated unwinding and re-rolling until a uniformly stretched microfiber web mesh is formed. This web is then acidified with phosphoric acid, to neutralize residual ionomer on the fibers, and water rinsed.

Freeze-Drying – The utility of the microfiber nonwoven fabric as a substrate for tissue growth is highly dependent upon its porosity. The surface fiber network must be sufficiently open to facilitate cellular infiltration. There must similarly be adequate three dimensional spacing within the microfiber web to accommodate cells and to permit adequate fluid circulation for their survival. At the same time, fiber packing should not be so low in density that adequate mechanical attachment of the intimal lining cannot be achieved.

The manner in which microfiber meshes are dried after formation by transverse drafting is a most significant factor in controlling porosity of the fabric's network. As initially formed, water-swollen microfiber meshes tend to be relatively thick and highly porous. If dried by evaporation in air, they are compacted in thickness and the density is correspondingly increased because of water's surface tension. To achieve a high porosity, it is necessary to employ freeze-drying techniques. The technique used starts with immersion of the water-swollen microfiber mesh, in rolled form, in n-hexane chilled to dry ice temperature. The frozen water is then removed from the microfiber roll by sublimation under a vacuum of less than 1 mm Hg (1 torr). Since the water remains frozen during drying, the microfiber web retains in the dry state and depth and porosity of the swollen material before freezing. Scanning electron micrographs (SEM) of microfiber webs prepared by freeze-drying indicate that these samples are many times deeper and more porous than equivalent samples dried by evaporation. If webs prepared by freeze-drying are reswollen in water and then redried by evaporation, they are converted to the more dense form. However, once conformally coated with parylene C (as described later), freeze-dried microfiber webs retain their porosity, even if immersed in water and then air dried.

Tentering – A small increase in porosity can be achieved by tentering freeze-dried microfiber webs. This is done by gently pulling the dry microfiber web in the original machine direction. In the dry state, a freeze-dried web can be tentered to increase its width 2 to 3-fold. Although the web becomes slightly thinner and more porous as a result of this procedure, the main advantages are in improved uniformity. Small areas in which microfibers are closely packed will pull out to a porosity about equal to that of the remainder of the web. In addition, wrinkles and puckers in the ultrathin fabric are also smoothed out.

Parylene Coating — At this point a very light coating (<1500 Å) of parylene C is applied to the microfiber fabric to facilitate its handling. Parylene is also a vital part of the subsequent microfiber lining process.

The solution to the problem of biocompatibility and network reinforcement depended upon utilization of the unusual properties of parylene polymers. The application of commercial parylene polymers (such as parylene C) requires a license from Union Carbide Corporation. In addition to having excellent biocompatibility, impermeability, and chemical stability, the parylene polymers owe their uniqueness to the process by which they are formed and the resultant nature of the thin parylene coating. In the vacuum polymerization process, cyclic p-xylylene dimer converted to the reactive monomer, p-xylylene. Condensation of the monomer vapor on cool (room temperature) substrate surfaces is followed by immediate polymerization to poly (p-xylylene). A continuous adherent coating is formed which precisely replicates all contours of the surface.

Because of the conformal nature of the parylene coating, vapor deposition onto a fiber web results in the encapsulation of each individual fiber in a parylene sheath, as well as the formation of a continuous parylene film at the surface of the adhesive on the backing (Figure 1). By keeping the parylene layer thin relative to the interfiber distance, parylene deposition also provides fiber-to-backing and fiber-to-fiber bonding without significantly decreasing pore size. A parylene C coating of about 0.5 micron total thickness is normally employed to provide substantial fiber web reinforcement.

Types of Test Devices and Microfiber Linings. Four main styles of test devices have been supplied for biological evaluation — tissue culture rings and discs, aortic tube grafts, and blood pump bladders. Microfiber linings exist in three principal types — B (nonvertically drafted); E (vertically drafted Type B); Composite. While their application and microfiber lining procedures depend upon the type of test devices, they all employ an elastomer adhesive for attaching the lining to the device backing surface. The adhesive, specially developed by us for this purpose, is a dope

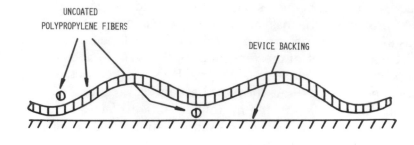

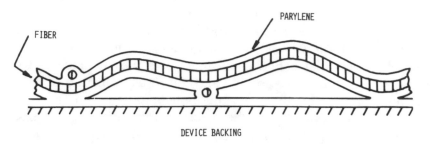

Figure 1. Parylene C vapor deposition onto microfiber lining
(Cross-sectional diagram).

solution of polyurethane, dimethylformamide solvent, and a commercial pressure sensitive adhesive (Ashland Chemical Co., No. A-1160). It is applied by brush to the backing surface upon which the microfiber lining is bonded.

Microfiber Linings — ● Type B [2,12] linings (Figures 2a,b) consist of the dual microfiber networks originating from tubular lay-flat laminated film. The linings, while possessing good density and cellular adhesion, do not have adequate physical integrity to withstand the rigors of long-term repeated flexure and stretching, such as is required for a bladder. The bottom layer can have satisfactory attachment to the wall, but the upper web may eventually separate at various spots and cause microfiber lining blebs.

● Type E [2,12] has better network porosity and flex behavior than Type B. Cell growth is more readily encouraged in static testing, either in vitro or in vivo. However, because of the lower density of the fibers network, cellular adhesion under repeated flexure is inferior to Type B. The microfiber lining is made from Type B by a delayering technique which

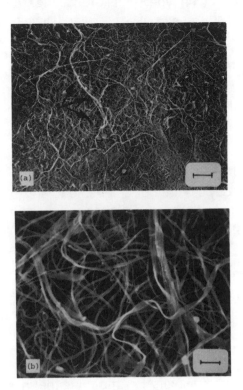

Figure 2. SEM of (a) lining Type B, 100×.
Bar = 100 μm, (b) 10× magnification of figure 2a
(Arrow Region). Bar = 10μm.

we have named "vertical drafting." This is a procedure by which freeze-dried and tentered microfiber webs can be opened into random networks in which the strata nearest the surface contain extremely large pores. It is done after the microfabric has been bonded to the device backing.

Vertical drafting entails removing the upper free surface of the fabric by peeling it away from the lower portion. As the two layers are pulled apart, fibers are drawn from the fabrics and ultimately fracture to form separate microfiber layers on both of the parted surfaces. Vertical drafting produces a highly porous surface layer which can be readily infiltrated by cells. It also creates large voids between the highly porous surface network and the less porous web beneath it. These voids are large enough to accommodate cells able to penetrate the upper layer.

● The *composite* [11,14] type is a tailored lining structure, designed to have the combined advantages of types E and B linings, and without their faults. It provides blood pump bladder microfiber linings having a balance of density, for suitable cellular adhesion, against good physical integrity under long-term repeated flexure. The composite is built-up on the device surface in two separate fibrous web layers, each vertically drafted after lay-up. The bottom layer is very lightly coated (<1500 Å) with parylene C, and a thin adhesive solution of A-1160 in isopropyl alcohol applied for bonding the top layer. Parylene C overcoating of this complete provides additional coherence and bonding of the network.

Test Devices – The rings, discs [2,12] and aortic grafts [11,14] are made by us. Since these devices are not amenable to steam sterilization, they are heat sealed in polyethylene envelopes and radiation sterilized before shipment. Radiation treatment is 5 megarads using a Van de Graaf electron accelerator.

● Rings and discs are flat devices fabricated as culture holders for *in vitro* evaluation. Lining types B, E, or composite are available. Ring devices have straight-walled cylindrical cavities. They are made starting with microfabric bonded to 0.013 mm thick polyurethane film, solution cast on 0.13 mm gauge polypropylene sheet. A ring is formed by attaching the sheet with elastomer adhesive on the microfiber covered side to a high density polyethylene ring (1.4 mm thick × 25 mm OD with a 16 mm diameter center opening). After trimming the sheet to size, the dish is parylene C overcoated and glow discharge treated. Disc devices (16 mm diameter) are made from microfabric bonded and parylene C overcoated on 0.5 mm thick plaques of compression molded high modulus polyurethane. These discs are cut out with a die and glow discharge treated.

● Aortic grafts have been used for either *in vivo* or tissue' culture studies. The tubes are seamless walled (20 mm OD × 50 mm long) injection molded polyurethane [B.F. Goodrich Estane 5714-F1; an unfilled ether polyurethane, modulus of 1.03×10^7 Nm^{-2} (1500 psi)]. A tube blank is lined from within after solvent cleaning and adhesive coating the inside surface. It is slightly enlarged in diameter on an expansible mandrel and frozen in dry ice. The rigidified tube is then removed and slipped over microfabric which has been laid up on a similar mandrel, and smoothed by expanding. The tube contracts during warming to its original diameter and adheres to the microfiber web. A 90 mm long Dacron velour sleeve of USCI noncrimped vascular prosthesis material is slipped over the lined tube, and bonded with elastomer adhesive to both exterior ends of the tube. The sleeve is folded back over the tube body to form a 3 mm extension, or sewing cuff, for anastomosis of the tube to the aorta. The lined tube and sleeve asembly are parylene C coated and glow discharge treated. Either types B or E linings are available.

● The *blood pump bladder* [11,14] is an open-ended axisymmetric pear shaped piece. Manufactured by TECO, it is their Model 10 Tecothane B bladder for the bypass pumping chamber of LVAD systems. It is intended for *in vivo* clinical and animal studies. The bladder lining approach used is a lay-up of the microfabric over an everted bladder. Composite linings are normally made. The bladder is first turned inside out and mounted over a silicone rubber collapsible "Chinese puzzle" mandrel having the Model 10 inside configuration. The exposed bladder surface is solvent cleaned and painted with elastomer adhesive after which both microfabric layers are laid up, each in two halves with seamed overlaps. After parylene C coating, the mandrel is removed and the bladder reinverted. The outer surface is masked, and the lining is parylene C overcoated followed by glow discharge treatment.

Biological Evaluation Procedures

Tissue culture studies with both non- and vertically drafted microfiber materials were initially carried out by the following investigator groups. Their work has been reported [2-5,12]:

● Dr. J. Boatman and coworkers at Battelle Memorial Institute, Columbus, Ohio.

● Dr. R. Kahn and coworkers at University of Michigan (UM), Ann Arbor, Michigan [10].

● Dr. P. Mansfield and coworkers at the Reconstructive Cardiovascular Research Center (RCR) of Providence Medical Center, Seattle, Washington.

More recently, ongoing extensive testing of microfiber materials has been conducted by Dr. Mansfield's group. The microfiber materials underwent a uniform sequence of evaluation, both *in vitro* as substrates for tissue culture cell linings, and in calves as the surfaces of implanted aortic grafts and Model 10 pump bladders. The detailed methods of seeding, culturing, shear testing, and histological preparation of the microfiber lined ring specimens and grafts together with results have been described [4,5,8]. Corresponding studies with the pump bladders were started within the past several years and have been reported [7,11].

Dr. Eskin and coworkers at Baylor College of Medicine (BCM), Houston, Texas also have been carrying out cell culture studies since 1976 with microfiber linings, both *in vitro* and on atrial implant patches in calves [6.9].

BIOLOGICAL PERFORMANCE OF MICROFIBER LININGS

Evaluation results from calf implants and *in vitro* tests of microfiber lined devices precultured with autologous endothelial cells have established microfiber material as a usable scaffolding for achieving compatibility with blood contacting surfaces in artificial vascular and cardiac prostheses.

RCR's *in vitro* evaluation of types B, E, and composite microfiber linings found these to support uniform cell linings. Shear tests [3,4,14] showed more extensive cell necrosis with Type E than types B or composite. The latter had slightly more fabric disruption than Type B. These results correlate with calf implantations of aortic grafts having cultured types B and E microfiber linings, and also in pump bladders having composite linings [3,4,14]. *In vivo* studies of both uncultured and cultured endothelial prelined bladders using composite type microfibers have been conducted in a series of eleven calves [7,11,15]. Seven of these bladders were precultured. Their implantation times ranged from several hours to seven days. The four uncultured controls went for three days and longer periods (30, 60, and 132 days). The precultured samples were found to inhibit thrombus formation and encourage endothelial cell growth. Some separation of microfiber lining from the bladder backing was observed in both sets of samples tested beyond three days. This problem has prompted our further investigation of means to achieve improved microfiber bonding.

The experimental work of RCR provides an insight to the mode of cellular lining formation after implantation *in vivo* [15]. Cells proliferate within the interstices of the microfiber network during the *in vitro* culture period. However, following implantation *in vivo*, the cultured cell lining thins to a single layer. The cells become greatly elongated, bridge the microfibers and form a continuous covering on the superficial surface of the fabric. No cells are then seen intertwining with individual microfibers. Proliferation beneath the surface layer appears to be neither necessary nor desirable.

The results of BCM's studies, while limited to atrial patches, have also demonstrated that cultured endothelial cell linings supported by microfiber substrates may inhibit thrombus formation following implantation. The relationship between microfiber material and growing endothelial cells is depicted in Figure 3. The microfibers are surrounded by the cytoplasm, as if the cells were attempting to phagocytose the material, in contrast to the poorer growth pattern with Dacron [9,16]. Figure 4 is from earlier studies at UM [10,12,17] and shows the cell microvilli attachment to the microfibers.

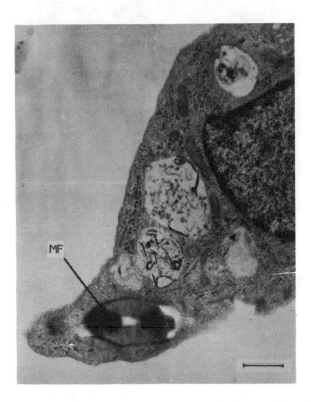

Figure 3. Transmission electron micrograph showing the relationship between the atrial patch microfabric (MF) and an endothelial cell. Bar = 2 μm (Photo courtesy of Dr. S.G. Eskin, et al., [9,16].

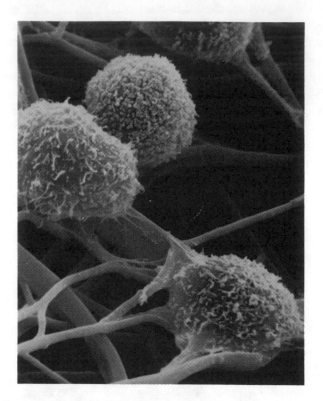

Figure 4. Sem of type B lining on culture disc seeded with human epidermal cells, fixed for microscopy about 15 minutes later: original approximately 6000×. (Photo courtesy of Dr. W.E. Burkel [17], Sample No. 20794; Union Carbide Specimen No. B9863-45-72).

FUTURE WORK

Our present solutions to the fabrication problem areas discussed are not ideal. But they have been satisfactory enough to enable implantation of microfiber lined devices and demonstrating blood compatibility and feasibility of the scaffolding approach system. Improved microfiber structures and fabrication techniques will be tried. Progress in the development of these or candidate new materials will rely heavily on future feedback from biological investigators. Cooperation between them and our biomaterial engineers at the planning stages of microfabric development will also be of benefit.

REFERENCES

1. Brash, J.L., Keller, K.H., LaFarge, G., Mason, R.G., Pierce, W.S., Reynolds, J.A., Galletti, P.M. Report of the Task Force on Biomaterials to the Cardiology Advisory Committee, NHLBI, January 1978.
2. Miller, W.A., Spivack, M.A., Tittmann, F.R., and Byck, J.S. Ultrathin Microfiber Lining for Artificial Organs (Paper presented at Fiber Society Symposium in New York City, N.Y., October 1971). Manuscript Reprinted in Textile Research Journal, *43:* December 1973, 728-734.
3. Mansfield, P.B., Tissue Cultured Endothelium for Vascular Prosthetic Devices. Annual Report No. NIH-NHLI 71-2060-2, Division of Technological Applications, National Heart and Lung Institute, NIH, Bethesda, Maryland, 1973.
4. Mansfield, P.B., Tissue Cultured Endothelium for Vascular Prosthetic Devices. Annual Reort No. NIH-NHLI 71-2060-3 and 71-2060-4, Devices and Technology Branch, Division of Heart and Vascular Diseases, National Heart and Lung Institute, NIH, Bethesda, Maryland, 1975.
5. Mansfield, P.B., Wechezak, A.R., and Sauvage, L.R., Preventing Thrombus of Artificial Vascular Surfaces: True Endothelial Cell Linings. Trans. Amer. Soc. Artif. Int. Organs, *21:* 1975, 264-272.
6. Eskin, S.G., Trevino, L., Aortic Endothelial Cells and Smooth Muscle Cells Cultured on Cardiovascular Biomaterials. Scanning Electron Microscopy, Part V, 1976, 209-216.
7. Mansfield, P.B. and Wechezak, A.R., Tissue Cultured Endothelium for Vascular Prosthetic Devices. Contractor Conference Program, Devices and Technology Branch, Division of Heart and Vascular Diseases, National Heart, Lung, and Blood Institute, NIH, Bethesda, Maryland, December 1977.
8. Mansfield, P.B., Wechezak, A.R., DiBenedetto, G., and Sauvage, L.R., Antithrombogenic Functions of the Endothelium. *Vascular Grafts* (Ed. Phillip N. Sawyer and Martin J. Kaplitt), 1978, 130-146, Appleton-Century Crofts, New York.
9. Eskin, S.G., Sybers, H.D., and Trevino, L., Thromboresistant Surfaces of Tissue Cultured Endothelial Cells. Scanning Electron Microscopy, *2:* 1978, 747-754.
10. Burkel, W.E. and Kahn, R.H., Cell-Lined, Nonwoven Microfiber Scaffolds as a Blood Interface. Annals of the New York Academy of Sciences, *283:* February 10, 1977, 419-442.
11. Beach, W.F. and Tittmann, F.R., Microfiber Materials for Growth of Initial Linings in Circulatory Assist Devices. Annual Report NO1-HV-8-1388-A7, Devices and Technology Branch, Division of Heart and Vascular Diseases, National Heart, Lung, and Institute, NIH, Bethesda, Maryland, 1978.
12. Byck, J.S., Barth, B.P., Gaasch, J.F., Miller, W.A., Stewart, D.D., and Tittmann, F.R., Microfiber materials for Growth of Intimal Linings in Circulatory Assist Devices Applications Program, National Heart and Lung Institute, NIH, Bethesda, Maryland, 1972.
13. Harris, A. Behavior of Cultured Cells: Variable Adhesiveness. Exp. Cell Res., *77:* 1973, 285-297.
14. Beach, W.F. and Tittmann, F.R., Microfiber Materials for Growth of Intimal Linings in Circulatory Assist Devices. Annual Report NO1-HV-8-1388-A4, Devices and Technology Branch, Division of Heart and Vascular Diseases, National Heart and Lung Institute, NIH, Bethesda, Maryland, 1975.
15. Wechezak, A.R., Personal Communication, 1978.
16. Eskin, S.G., Personal Communication, 1978.
17. Burkel, W.E., Personal Communication, 1978.

SURFACE GRAFTED POLYMERS FOR BIOMEDICAL APPLICATIONS

Buddy D. Ratner and Allan S. Hoffman

*Department of Chemical Engineering
and
Center for Bioengineering
University of Washington
Seattle, Washington 98195*

ABSTRACT

Surface grafting techniques are useful for preparing new polymers for use as biomaterials, and for modifying the surface properties of existing polymers. The techniques for the preparation of graft polymers are reviewed. Methods for characterization of graft polymers, particularly gravimetric techniques, thermodynamic measurements, surface chemistry characterization, and topographic characterization, are summarized. The use of graft polymers as models for exploring the effect of surface free energy on biological interactions is described, and criteria for the development of polymeric model systems are outlined. The application of radiation grafting to the modification of porous Dacron arterial prostheses is discussed.

KEY WORDS

Grafted Polymers; Radiation Grafting; Surface Characterization; Domain Formation; Poly(2-hydroxyethyl methacrylate); Poly(ethyl methacrylate); Polyacrylamide; Cell Adhesion; Protein Adsorption; Hydrophilic/Hydrophobic; Arterial Prosthesis.

133

INTRODUCTION

Grafting Polymer Surfaces

The use of polymeric materials in biomedical applications is widespread. Since it is the surface of these materials which first contacts the biological environment, it is useful and important both to characterize as well as to control the surface state of the biomaterials before and after contact with biomolecules and cells.

Over the past 10 years, many researchers have investigated a variety of different techniques for chemical and biochemical modification of polymer surfaces, in order to render these surfaces more biologically compatible or even biologically active. In general, polymer surfaces may be modified chemically by:

(1) direct treatment with the modifying chemical system only (e.g., via polymerization, oxidation, hydrolysis, sulfonation, quaternization, etc.), or by

(2) pre-activation of the polymer surface with an energy source of chemical, electrochemical, mechanical, thermal, electromagnetic or high energy particle character, followed by contact with the modifying chemical system, or by

(3) activation of the surface with such an energy source in the presence of the modifying chemical system, or by

(4) direct treatment with the energy source only.

Table 1. Radiation Source Frequencies.

SOURCE	FREQUENCY Hz (cycles/sec)
Cosmic Rays	$> 10^{22}$
Gamma Rays	3×10^{19} to 10^{22}
X-rays	3×10^{16} to 3×10^{10}
Ultraviolet	10^{15} to 3×10^{16}
Visible	5×10^{14} to 10^{15}
Infrared	10^{12} to 5×10^{14}
Microwaves	10^{9} to 10^{12}
Radiofrequency	2×10^{5} to 10^{9}

For methods 2 to 4, the most commonly used energy sources involve electromagnetic or particulate radiations. The frequencies of some common radiation sources are listed in Table 1. This review will be particularly concerned with methods 1–3 where a surface is chemically activated and then contacted with a reactive chemical, usually a monomer, to form a graft modified surface.

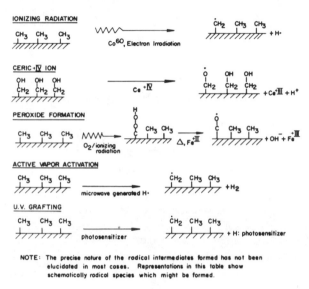

NOTE: The precise nature of the radical intermediates formed has not been elucidated in most cases. Representations in this table show schematically radical species which might be formed.

Figure 1. Examples of techniques and reactions for generating radicals on surfaces.

Many of the energy sources used for the modification of surfaces operate via atom or free radical reaction mechanisms. Figure 1 presents some schematic examples of how such species may be generated on polymer surfaces. If a monomer is present in contact with such free radical activated surfaces a polymerization reaction will be initiated in the surface regions resulting in a covalently bound graft.

Ionizing radiations for surface activation are commercially available as cobalt-60 gamma ray sources or as electron accelerators. The former are low intensity sources but have high depth of penetration while the latter are high intensity sources but have relatively low depth of penetration. Figure 2 compares these two (along with X-ray sources) in the dose range often needed to modify polymer surfaces.

Electric discharges may be classified as "cold," non-equilibrium plasmas or "hot," equilibrium plasmas. Some of the characteristics of these

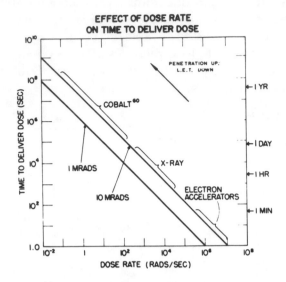

Figure 2. Effect of dose rate on time required to deliver 1 or 10 Mrad. doses, for radiation of different penetration abilities.

Table 2. Types of Electric Discharges.

Type	Pressure (torr)	Exit Plasma Character
Silent Discharge (e.g. Ozonizer)	760	"Cold", Non-Equilibrium
D.C. Glow Discharge	<100	"Cold", Non-Equilibrium
H.F. Glow Discharge	<100	"Cold", Non-Equilibrium
Arc Discharge-Plasma Torch	760	"Hot", Equilibrium

discharges are shown in Table 2. Electric discharges may also produce thermal and U.V. radiation, in addition to energetic electrons and ions, atoms and radicals.

Processes for preparing surface grafted polymers have the following steps in common. A surface is exposed to ionizing radiation, electric discharge or modified by chemical reaction producing reactive species (e.g., free radicals) at the surface. If monomer is present simultaneously with this surface activation, polymer chains will begin to propagate from the reactive sites. If the monomer is in liquid form, two simultaneous processes can occur; grafting and homopolymerization. Homopolymerization, the formation of polymer which is not covalently immobilized to the substrate polymer, depletes available monomer thereby reducing graft levels at the substrate. Excessive homopolymerization, particularly where branching and crosslinking reactions can take place, is troublesome since the graft polymer is often encapsulated in an intractable gel at the completion of the reaction. A number of ionic compounds have been found to be effective at reducing homopolymerization without retarding graft polymerization. The dramatic effect of cupric ion at reducing homopolymerization while allowing graft polymerization is illustrated in Table 3. Alternatively, the activated polymer can be removed from the activating agent and then later placed in contact with monomer. If oxygen is present, peroxides and hydroperoxides may form at the free radical sites; these can be activated later in the presence of monomer to initiate the graft reaction.

Table 3. Effect of $Cu(NO_3)_2$ on Cobalt 60 initiated Radiation Grafting on to Silicone Rubber (0.25 Mrad. dose) [1].

Monomer 1[a]	Monomer 2[a]	Solvent (80%)	Extent of graft, mg/cm²	H_2O in graft, %
2-Hydroxyethyl acrylate (10%)	N-VP (10%)	H_2O[b]	0	—
2-Hydroxyethyl acrylate (10%)	N-VP (10%)	$0.005M$ $Cu(NO_3)_2$	13.3	57.5
Acrylamide (10 g)	N-VP (10 g)	H_2O[b]	0	—
Acrylamide (10 g)	N-VP (10 g)	$0.005M$ $Cu(NO_3)_2$	2.5	60.2
Acrylamide (10 g.)	HEMA (10 g)	H_2O[b]	2.3	52.0
Acrylamide (10 g)	HEMA (10 g)	$0.005M$ $Cu(NO_3)_2$	2.7	46.3
Acrylamide (20 g)	—	H_2O[b]	0	—
Acrylamide (20 g)	—	$0.005M$ $Cu(NO_3)_2$	1.3	68.0
Propylene glycol acrylate (10%)	N-VP (10%)	H_2O[b]	0	—
Propylene glycol acrylate (10%)	N-VP (10%)	$0.005M$ $Cu(NO_3)_2$	9.6	54.2
Methacrylamide (10 g)	N-VP (10 g)	H_2O[b]	8.1	62.9
Methacrylamide (10 g)	N-VP (10 g)	$0.005M$ $Cu(NO_3)_2$	4.2	60.5
Methacrylamide (5 g)	N-VP (15 g)	H_2O[b]	6.8	66.2
Methacrylamide (5 g)	N-VP (15 g)	$0.005M$ $Cu(NO_3)_2$	5.2	66.2

[a] Volume per cent or weight.
[b] External solution was found to be gelled after irradiation.

The final process in preparing graft polymers involves a thorough extraction with a good solvent for the homopolymer and monomer. This extraction solvent should be a non-solvent for the substrate and graft polymer. However, a good swelling solvent for the graft polymer and substrate will speed up complete extraction of unwanted, non-covalently bound material.

There are a number of advantages in using grafting techniques for preparing biomaterials. If the grafting is localized at the surface region of the substrate, the mechanical properties of the graft polymer will resemble those of the substrate; this is particularly useful when attempting to use mechanically weak polymers such as hydrogels for biomedical applications. The washing procedures necessary for preparing graft polymers should also remove all leachable compounds which might complicate the biological response to an implanted material. Using successive graftings, copolymer grafts which would be difficult to produce by solution copolymerization techniques can be prepared. Finally, by manipulating a variety of variables, a wide range of different types of graft polymers can be produced. Table 4 lists some of the variables which can be used to control the properties of radiation grafted polymers.

Table 4. Parameters Affecting the Properties of Radiation Grafted Polymers.

---

(1) Monomer system

    (a) purity

    (b) physical interaction with substrate polymer

    (c) monomer mixture composition (for copolymer grafts)

    (d) reactivity of the monomer (kinetics of polymerization,
        chain transfer, crosslink formation, and monomer "G-value")

(2) Solvent system

    (a) solubility of the polymerized monomer (homopolymer) in
        the solvent

    (b) interaction of the solvent with the substrate polymer

    (c) chain transfer by the solvent

    (d) radiolysis products of solvents (also "G-value")

(3) Support polymer

    (a) Interaction with radiation ("G-value")

    (b) Crystallinity

    (c) Chemical composition

    (d) Thickness

    (e) Fabrication method

(4) Radiation source, dose and dose rate

(5) Temperature during irradiation

(6) Atmosphere (presence or absence of O_2) during irradiation

Surface Characterization

Some of the most significant advances which have been made in the biomaterials field over the past ten years have been related to the application of surface characterization techniques to biomaterials problems. The true significance, in a scientific sense, of much of the biological evaluation of materials which was performed prior to this period is lost because the materials used were described only by a generic name or a trade name. As an example, the 1958 text, "Modern Trends in Surgical Materials," describes the method for obtaining materials for porous fabric prostheses as follows: "The Terylene, Orlon, or nylon cloth is bought from a draper's shop and cut with pinking shears to the desired shape. It is then sewn with thread of similar materials into a tube and sterilized by autoclaving before use." Without an intimate knowledge of the surface structure and properties of biomaterials, correlations between the physical nature of the implant and the biological response are impossible.

Often, the surface composition of a material can be significantly different from its bulk composition since the surface may be susceptible to chemical reaction, concentration of diffusable materials or polymer chain orientation effects related to fabrication or structure. For graft polymers in which the surface region is entirely different from the bulk, a thorough characterization of the surface is particularly important.

Four general categories of characterization techniques which are particularly applicable to graft polymers can be described:

Gravimetric Techniques
"Thermodynamic" Measurements
Surface Chemistry Characterization
Topographic Characterization

Specific surface characterization techniques, and the information which can be obtained from them are described in Tables 5, 6, 7, and 8.

An additional problem in surface characterization relating to both the surface chemistry and topography is that of domain formation. The spatial arrangement of regions of differing chemistry has received little attention in biomaterials studies. Yet the size of domains seen in some polymer system is often of the same order of magnitude as the end radius of the processes which extend from cells during their initial contact phase with foreign surfaces. Flexible chain segments and rigid, crystallizable chain segments have often been observed to organize

Table 5. Information Obtained from Gravimetric Analysis of Graft Polymers.

1) Extent of reaction (level of graft)

2) Proximity of graft to the surface (see figure 3)

3) Graft equilibrium water content

4) Extraction of leachable components

5) Macroporosity (see reference 2)

6) Surface coverage (see reference 3)

Table 6. Techniques for the Analysis of the Thermodynamic Properties of Grafted Polymer Surfaces.

(A) Contact angle measurements as an approximation of overall surface free energy

    1) Zisman technique [4]

    2) Hamilton technique [5]

    3) Kaelble method (γ_ρ γ_d determination) [6]

(B) Gas or Vapor Sorption Methods

    1) Surface area (BET method) (for large surface areas only)

    2) ΔH sorption, ΔG sorption, ΔS sorption [7, 8]

    3) Clustering function (e.g. of water) [8, 9]

    4) Diffusivity in the polymer [10]

Table 7. Surface Chemistry Characterization.

TECHNIQUE	PENETRATION DEPTH	CAPABILITIES
Attenuated Total Reflectance Infrared Spectrophotometry (ATR) [10]	~1 mμ	IR spectrum of surface region
Electron Spectroscopy for Chemical Analysis (ESCA) [11]	10 - 90 Å	Identify any element (Z>2) at surface. Determine oxidation state of elements Determine electronic environment (particularly C, N, O) Quantitative analysis Valence band spectra Depth profiling
Auger Electron Spectroscopy (AES) [11]	10 - 90 Å	Identify any element (Z>2) at surface. Spatially resolved elemental analysis ($\geq 2.5 \times 10^{-3}$mμ^2) Depth profiling

Table 8. Surface Topography Evaluation.

	Resolution
Stylus Techniques [12]	25Å
Scanning Electron Microscopy	35Å
Transmission Electron Microscopy (replica techniques)	10Å
Light Microscopy [13]	
(a) Interference Contrast Optics	1mμ
(b) Interferometric microscope	1mμ
(c) Stereo microscope	10mμ

themselves into domains at the surface of polyetherurethanes and other block copolymers. In addition, domain structure has been observed in hydrophilic/hydrophobic methacrylic networks [14] and even in homogeneous hydrogels [14].

Domain structures can be characterized by a variety of techniques. Specific staining methods use heavy metal "stains" which react with only one portion of the polymer surface. The surface can be "mapped" by using electron microscopic techniques or energy dispersive x-ray analysis. The surface can also be chemically etched to remove a small portion of only one type of surface structure. Etched surfaces can be examined by replica techniques using transmission electron microscopy. Other techniques which have been used to examine domain structures include ^{13}C NMR [14], light scattering [15], and differential scanning calorimetry [16].

GRAFT POLYMER SYSTEMS FOR BIOMEDICAL APPLICATIONS

Copolymer Graft Systems as Polymeric Models

By systematically varying the surface structure of materials and observing the effects of this variation on biological interactions, one can explore fundamental aspects of such phenomena as protein adsorption, cell adhesion, and thrombogenesis on foreign surfaces. Polymeric materials prepared specifically as model surfaces for studying biointeractions have not been utilized in most biomaterials investigations. In many studies, investigators have compared such diverse materials as Teflon or paraffin to cellophane or glass in order to determine the effects of wettability on biological interactions. Although highly wettable and non-wettable materials are being compared in these studies, the chemistry and surface structure of the surface property extremes are also entirely different. Therefore, it is difficult to attribute observed responses only to wettability.

Properly designed model systems can be used to explore surface wettability, surface charge, and surface chemistry. Five conditions should be satisfied by carefully designed polymeric model systems:

(1) The extremes should be structurally related. Examples of model systems which have common polymeric backbones are shown in Table 9.

Table 9. Polymer Series for Exploring Biological Phenomena.

Hydrophilic → Hydrophobic	$\{CH_2 - \underset{\underset{OCH_2CH_2OH}{\overset{\overset{CH_3}{\mid}}{\underset{C=0}{\mid}}}{C}\}_n$ p - HEMA	→	$\{CH_2 - \underset{\underset{OCH_2CH_3}{\overset{\overset{CH_3}{\mid}}{\underset{C=0}{\mid}}}{C}\}_n$ p - Ethyl Methacrylate
	$\{CH_2 - \underset{\underset{NH_2}{\underset{C=0}{\mid}}}{CH}\}_n$ p - Acrylamide	→	$\{CH_2 - \underset{\underset{N(C_4H_9)_2}{\underset{C=0}{\mid}}}{CH}\}_n$ p - N,N di-n-butyl Acrylamide
Neutral → Anionically Charged	$\{CH_2 - \underset{\underset{OCH_2CH_2OH}{\overset{\overset{CH_3}{\mid}}{\underset{C=0}{\mid}}}{C}\}_n$ P - HEMA	→	$\{CH_2 - \underset{\underset{OH}{\overset{\overset{CH_3}{\mid}}{\underset{C=0}{\mid}}}{C}\}_n$ p - Methacrylic Acid
Neutral → Cationically Charged	$\{CH_2 - \underset{\underset{OCH_2CH_2OH}{\overset{\overset{CH_3}{\mid}}{\underset{C=0}{\mid}}}{C}\}_n$ p - HEMA	→	$\{CH_2 - \underset{\underset{OCH_2CH_2N(CH_3)_2}{\overset{\overset{CH_3}{\mid}}{\underset{C=0}{\mid}}}{C}\}_n$ p - N,N dimethyl-aminoethyl methacrylate
Aliphatic → Aromatic	$\{CH_2 - \underset{\underset{OCH_2CH_3}{\underset{C=0}{\mid}}}{CH}\}_n$ p - Ethyl Acrylate	→	$\{CH_2 - \underset{\bigcirc}{CH}\}_n$ p - Styrene

(2) Polymer series used for such experimental studies should contain both the extremes (pure polymers) and a number of copolymers which are intermediate in properties to the extremes. If only the extremes are observed, maxima or minima in biological response as a function of composition might be missed; unexpected maxima or minima are frequently more revealing of the nature of the processes occurring than is a comparison of the extremes.

(3) More than one series covering a given property range should be used. If two structurally different hydrophilic-hydrophobic series are studied (e.g., methacrylic esters and acrylic amides, see Table 9), and both show similar variation in biological response as a function of composition, one might feel more secure in attributing the biological trend to hydrophilic-hydrophobic variation as opposed to some specific structural or chemical property of each series.

(4) The surfaces should be thoroughly characterized both macroscopically and microscopically. Techniques for performing such characterization are discussed in the second section of this review.

(5) The polymers used for studying biological interactions should be free of leachable components since these could complicate interpretation of responses induced by the surface.

Graft polymers are well suited for preparing model systems which satisfy the five criteria outlined above. Sufficient mechanical strength for evaluation is provided by a strong substrate polymer thus permitting the use of a much wider range of surface properties than would otherwise be possible. Also leachable components from graft polymer systems are usually removed during the extractive washing which is necessary to free the graft polymer from ungrafted polymer and monomers.

A graft polymer system which we have developed to explore the relationships between surface hydrophilicity and various biological phenomena is the hydroxyethyl methacrylate (HEMA)-ethyl methacrylate (EMA) copolymer system [2]. Grafts on silicone rubber, polyethylene and polyurethane consisting of HEMA polymer, EMA polymer and up to 9 different copolymers have been prepared (Figure 3). The variation in equilibrium water content as a function of composition for these systems is shown in Figure 4. Surface properties vary from highly wettable at the HEMA extreme to non-wettable for the EMA graft polymer. We have also used HEMA-EMA graft polymers to explore a variety of biological phenomena. In Figure 5 chick embryo myoblast cell adhesion to this

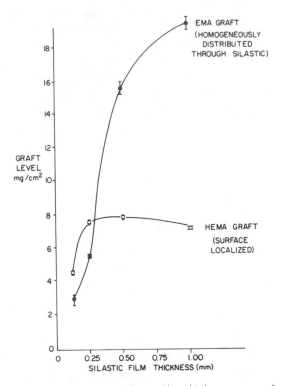

Figure 3. Effect of Silastic film thickness on graft level for hydroxyethyl methacrylate (HEMA) and ethyl methacrylate (EMA) radiation grafts (0.25 Mrad. dose).

series is described. A minimum in adhesion is noted as well as a sharp increase in adhesion occurring at a monomer ratio of approximately 1:1 [17]. A similar trend has been noted with these polymers for mouse erythrocyte adhesion in the absence of serum [18]. HEMA-EMA copolymers are found to be well suited for observing the effects of surface hydrophilicity on protein adosprtion from pure solution and from plasma [19]. A sharp maxima in fibrinogen adsorption has been found at intermediate HEMA-EMA copolymer compositions [20]. We are also studying the adhesion and morphology of primary fibroblasts, 3T3 fibroblasts, neutrophils, macrophages and platelets on this copolymer system.

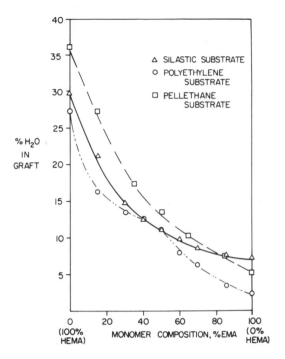

*Figure 4. Variation in equilibrium graft water con-
tent as a function of composition for HEMA/EMA
radiation graft copolymers on Silastic, polyethylene
and Pellethane.*

The development of a complimentary graft copolymer system to the
HEMA-EMA system, the acrylamide-N,N-di-n-butylacrylamide (NNDBA)
graft copolymer system, has been undertaken in order to further explore
the effects of surface hydrophilicity on cell and protein interactions. This
system should provide more information than has been obtained from
the HEMA-EMA graft polymers, since a wider range of graft water contents is covered (Figure 6).

We developed the hydrophilic-hydrophobic graft systems in order to
explore the effect of surface energy on cell and protein interactions with
surfaces. Although the chemistry of the backbone polymer is similar in
both systems for the hydrophilic and hydrophobic extremes, other
potentially important parameters are unavoidably changing as a function
of composition. Variables which must be considered include

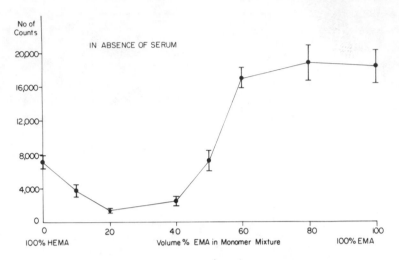

Figure 5. Adhesion of ³H labelled myoblast cells to HEMA/EMA graft polymers on silicone rubber.

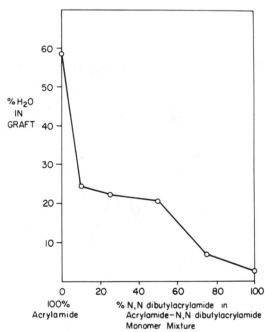

Figure 6. Equilibrium graft water content for acrylamide-N,N-dibutyl-acrylamide graft polymers on silicone rubber prepared using a 0.25 Mrad. radiation dose.

permeability, surface modulus, water content, wettability, specific functional group density (e.g., hydroxyl group density in the HEMA-EMA series), domain formation, and finally, the surface property which is of primary interest, surface free energy. Thus, although HEMA-EMA copolymers and acrylamide-NNDBA copolymers appear to be simple model systems for exploring hydrophilic-hydrophobic character, the interpretation of results can be complicated by the multi-variable nature of these systems. We are exploring another graft system to eliminate some of the objectionable aspects of the two previously mentioned systems. Copolymers of polystyrene and poly(p-hydroxystyrene) range from non-polar to polar in surface properties. However, all compounds in the series are essentially non-swelling in water, and, therefore, are all similar in modulus and permeability. If similarities are noted in biological response between all three systems, then general conclusions about the effect of polymer surface free energy on biological phenomena may be drawn.

A similar rationale to that presented above should apply to the development of neutral/charged systems for exploring biological phenomena. HEMA-methacrylic acid copolymers prepared as radiation grafts in series ranging electrostatically neutral to highly charged, have different water contents at physiological pH (Figure 7). Surface modulus and permeability will also vary within this series of graft compounds. A series of model polymer surfaces based upon carboxylated or sulfonated polystyrene should be of value for observing the effects of negatively charged surfaces since, for low degrees of carboxylation or sulfonation, the surface modulus and permeability should be relatively constant throughout the series.

Radiation Graft Modified Knitted Dacron Arterial Prostheses

The effect of surface composition in the *in vivo* healing of porous arterial and venous prostheses has never fully been evaluated. Although a wide variety of polymers including Dacron, Teflon, silicone rubber, polyurethane, polypropylene, and Nylon have been studied, the porosities of the different implants have always varied simultaneously with the fabric composition. Since porosity has been shown to be a critical variable with respect to the healing of arterial prostheses, it is impossible to draw conclusions as to the effect of surface composition on the healing process. However, by radiation graft treating the surfaces

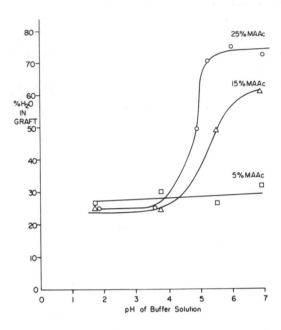

Figure 7. Equilibrium graft water content of radiation grafted films on silicone rubber prepared using solutions containing 25% methacrylic acid (MAAC)/75% HEMA, 15% MAAC/85% HEMA and 5% MAAC/95% HEMA after storage for 40 days in citric acid buffer solution.

of porous Dacron arterial prostheses, the healing response as a function of composition with essentially constant porosity and fabric geometry can be studied.

Radiation grafting to Dacron (polyethylene terephthalate) presents a number of problems. The aromatic ring structures in the polymer dissipate radiation resulting in low "G" values and consequently, a low grafting efficiency for the polymer. Also, the polymer is difficult to swell, thus usually restricting reaction to only the immediate surface regions. These problems have been overcome by grafting at elevated temperatures while using specific swelling solvents for the Dacron and larger radiation doses (up to 3/8 Mrad.). Figure 8 shows the effect of two swelling solvents on the level of graft on knitted Dacron fabric. Only a moderate increase in graft level is noted with cyclohexanone since this solvent inhibits grafting while simultaneously opening more sites for

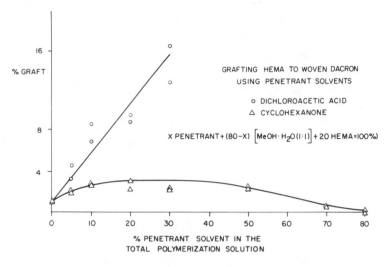

Figure 8. Radiation grafting of HEMA to Dacron fabric using penetrant solvents (0.375 Mrad. dose, ~70°C reaction temperature).

reaction by swelling the polymer. Dichloroacetic acid in methanol-water solutions is an effective swelling agent for Dacron and can be used to promote high levels of grafting. However, dichloroacetic acid is also a strong acid and may damage the polyethylene terephthate by hydrolytic mechanisms. Tetrachloroethane has also been found to be a highly effective grafting solvent for Dacron. Graft levels up to 50% at 3/8 Mrad. radiation dose are easily achieved without potential problems caused by hydrolysis of the Dacron fabric in strongly acidic solutions. Using this grafting solvent, HEMA/EMA grafts on knitted Dacron arterial prostheses have been prepared. These are being evaluated *in vivo* by implantation in dogs to assess the effect of polymer composition on healing at constant fabric porosity.

CONCLUSIONS

This review article presents an overview of graft polymer preparation for biomedical applications and of our program at the University of Washington directed towards the production of new biomaterials by graft polymerization techniques. This program has two fundamental components; the development of new biomaterials and devices, and the exploration of fundamental aspects of the interfacial interactions of biological systems with foreign interfaces. Our philosophy with respect to the development of new materials based upon graft polymerization reactions can be expressed by the statements:

(1) In order to understand the mechanisms of interaction of biological systems with foreign interfaces, a thorough knowledge of the structure and properties of those interfaces is essential.

(2) A systematic approach to exploring the interactions of well-characterized polymers with living systems must be adopted in order to minimize the number of variables which can complicate the interpretation of experimental results.

ACKNOWLEDGEMENT

Generous support for much of the work described in this article has been provided by U.S.E.R.D.A. contract NO. EY-76-S-06-2225T22 and N.H.L.B.I. grant No. HL19419-02. The authors also wish to acknowledge the valuable contributions of our collaborators, Dr. Thomas Horbett and Dr. Stephen Hauschka.

REFERENCES

1. Ratner, B.D., and Hoffman, A.S., "The Effects of Cupric Ion on the Radiation Grafting of N-vinyl-2-Pyrrolidone and Other Hydrophilic Monomers on Silicone Rubber," *J. Appl. Polym. Sci., 18,* 3183 (1974).

2. Sasaki, T., Ratner, B.D., and Hoffman, A.S., "Radiation Induced Co-graft Polymerization of 2-Hydroxyethyl Methacrylate and Ethyl Methacrylate onto Silicone Rubber Films," ACS Symposium Series, No. 31, J.D. Andrade, Editor, Washington, D.C., American Chemical Society, 283-294 (1976).

3. Ratner, B.D., and Hoffman, A.S., "Synthetic Hydrogels for Biomedical Applications," ACS Symposium Series, No. 31, J.D. Andrade, Editor, Washington, D.C., American Chemical Society, 1-36 (1976).

4. Zisman, W.A., "Relation of the Equilibrium Contact Angle to Liquid and Solid Constitution," ACS Advances in Chemistry Series No. 43, Washington, D.C., American Chemical Society, 1-51, (1964).

5. Hamilton, W.C., "A Technique for the Characterization of Hydrophilic Solid Surfaces," *J. Colloid. Interface Sci., 40,* 219 (1972).

6. Kaelble, D.H., "Dispersion-Polar Surface Tension Properties of Organic Solids," *J. Adhesion, 2,* 66 (1970).

7. Othmer, D.F., "Correlating Vapor Pressure and Latent Heat Data," *Ind. Eng. Chem.*, *32*, 841 (1940).
8. Khaw, B., Ratner, B.D., and Hoffman, A.S., "The Thermodynamics of Water Sorption in Radiation Grafted Hydrogels," ACS Symposium Series, No. 31, J.D. Andrade, Editor, Washington, D.C., American Chemical Society, 295-304 (1976).
9. Zimm, B.H. and Lundberg, J.L., "Sorption of Vapors by High Polymers," *J. Phys. Chem. 60*, 425 (1956).
10. Harrick, N.J., "Internal Reflection Spectroscopy," New York, Interscience, (1967).
11. Carlson, T.A., "Photoelectron and Auger Spectroscopy," New York, Plenum Press, (1975).
12. Whitehouse, D.J., "Stylus Techniques," "Characterization of Solid Surfaces," P.F. Kane and G.R. Larrabee, Editors, New York, Plenum Press, 49-74 (1974).
13. McCrone, W.C., "Light Microscopy," "Characterization of Solid Surfaces," P.F. Kane and G.R. Larrabee, Editors, New York, Plenum Press, 1-32 (1974).
14. Yokota, K., Abe, A., Hosaka, S., Sakai, I., and Saito, H., "A ^{13}C Nuclear Magnetic Resonance Study of Covalently Cross-linked Gels. Effect of Chemical Composition, Degree of Cross-linking and Temperature to Chain Mobility," *Macromolecules*, *11*(1), 95 (1978).
15 Donkersloot, M.C.A., Gouda, J.H., Van Aarsten, J.J., Prins, W., "Polymer Gel Structure Elucidation by Means of Light Scattering and Photo-elasticity," *Recueil, 86,* 321 (1967).
16. Seymour, R.W. and Cooper, S.L., "DSC Studies of Polyurethane Block Polymers," *Polymer Letters, 9*, 689 (1971).
17. Ratner, B.D., Hauschka, S.D., Horbett, T.A., Hoffman, A.S. and Rosen, J.J., "Cell Adhesion to Hydrophilic-Hydrophobic Copolymers," *Trans. 4th Annual Meeting, Soc. for Biomaterials, 2*, 64 (1978).
18. Horbett, T.A. and Ratner, B.D., unpublished results.
19. Weathersby, P.K., Horbett, T.A. and Hoffman, A.S., "Fibrinogen Adsorption to Surfaces of Varying Hydrophilicity," *J. Bioeng., 1,* 395 (1977).
20. Horbett, T.A., Weathersby, P.K., and Hoffman, A.S., "Plasma Protein Adsorption to a Series of Poly(Hydroxyethylmethacrylate-ethylmethacrylate) Copolymers," Abstracts of Papers — 51st Colloid and Surface Science Symposium, Grand Island, N.Y., 109 (1977).

FABRICATION AND CHARACTERIZATION OF GRAFTED HYDROGEL COATINGS AS BLOOD CONTACTING SURFACES*

Paul L. Kronick

The Franklin Institute Research Laboratories
Philadelphia, PA. 19103

ABSTRACT

Water-swollen synthetic polymers, or hydrogels, exhibit superior com-patibility with blood in vitro and ex vivo. It has been very difficult to prepare them, however, in a useful form which can be implanted into the vascular system in vivo. Because of their mechanical properties it appears that they can best be used as intravascular linings, applied as coatings on plastic substrata. Six techniques for achieving such coatings, with their physical and biological properties, are reviewed: simple adhesion, in-terpenetrating networks, chemical grafting with oxidizing solutions, non-ionizing irradiation, active-vapor methods, and radiation grafting.

KEY WORDS

Atomic hydrogen; blood; blood cells; clotting; fibrinogen; globulin; graft copolymerization; hydrogel grafts; hydrogels; hydrophilic surfaces; nonthrombogenic surfaces; platelets; polyacrylamide; polyetherure-thane; polypropylene; radiation grafting; renal-embolism test; silicone rubber; thrombogenic; 2-hydroxyethylmethacrylate; vascular implants; vena-cava test; vinyl pyrrolidone.

---

*Supported by NHLBI-NIH Contract No. NO1-HV-1-2017.

INTRODUCTION

It has been generally realized, since the beginning of a program under-taken by the U.S. National Heart, Lung, and Blood Institute in 1964 to develop a totally implanted artificial heart, that the tendency of blood to clot on foreign surfaces would be a major obstacle to the clinical use of such devices. It has been assumed for some time that, even after materials have been found that satisfy the mechanical and chemical re-quirements of artificial organs, they will have to be coated with something to make them compatible with blood. We find it easy to list 10 requirements for such coatings which, together, are very difficult to satisfy:

1. They must be nonthrombogenic.
2. They must resist physiological solutions, shearing forces, stretching, and swelling by lipids.
3. They must be applicable in thin layers.
4. No introduction of toxic reagents is permitted.
5. No introduction of solvents or swelling agents into substrata is per-mitted.
6. No excessive heating of substrata is permitted.
7. Reactants must be very fluid so that irregular surfaces (foams, fibers, and powders) can be coated.
8. Coatings must be uniform without holes, points, whiskers, or streamers.
9. The method of application must be adaptable to a variety of inert substrata and coating materials, since the first requirement, non-thrombogenicity, has never been satisfied by any synthetic material.
10. Good economic and technological feasibility for application to large surfaces, including dialysis and oxygenator membranes, blood-storage bags, and other mass-produced items.

The first requirement is best satisfied if the components of the blood, both solutes and formed elements, are indifferent to the presence of the foreign surface. Several thermodynamic criteria for such inert surfaces have been proposed. One possibility is that the free energy of adsorption of components of blood onto the surface should be zero or positive. Another is that the free energy for forming the interface between blood and the implant should be zero (otherwise the blood elements would tend to deposit on the surface to lower the area of the interface) [1]. It would appear that either conditions would be satisfied if the surface is chemically and physically similar to the aqueous solution. Therefore, water swollen polymers, hydrogels [2], are candidates for vascular-implant interfaces.

Polymers of many different types have been widely used for coatings in intravascular devices. Application of hydrogels as nonthrombogenic coatings, however, introduces problems which are peculiar to this type of material, related to their incompatibility with likely structural plastics for the devices, and to the difficulty in characterizing them locally in the coatings. Hydrogels are typically prepared from aqueous or very polar solvents, from which they ust be spread in thin films upon nonpolar substrata such as polypropylene, siicone, or polyetherurethane. Because the two phases, hydrophilic and hydrophobic, have little mutual affinity, the interface is unstable and adhesion is poor. For this reason special methods have been developed, which in some cases are rather elaborate, to effect a physical or chemical bond between the hydrogel coating and the substratum.

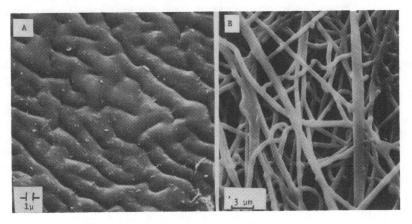

Figure 1. Surfaces graft coated with polyhydroxyethylmethacryate. A. The surface of polyetherurethane (3-1000/425-1-X(70/30), first swollen with monomer in a penetrating solvent, then polymerized at the surface by means of active-hydrogen initiation. "Hill and valley" effect due to differential swelling of the two layers. B. Polypropylene microfibrils surface grafted with vapors of hydroxyethylmethacrylate and atomic hydrogen.

After a hydrophobic surface has been coated with hydrogel, a composite structure results in which the two components swell differentially when equilibrated with water. The result is a potential mechanical instability (Figure 1), which may affect the performance of flexible parts such as pump diaphragms. Again, during the coating process, some components of thermoplastic substrata may migrate into the hydrogel layer, altering the nature of the hydrophilic product from that obtained in the absence of organic substrata. It is therefore necessary to analyze the chemical composition and the physical behavior of the coating *in situ*, even if it is only a few microns thick.

The use of hydrogels as nonthrombogenic surfaces is based on their low interfacial tension with water as pointed out above. This parameter is minimized at high water content of the gel. Therefore the surface coatings must be characterized by measurements of wetting angles as well as protein adsorption and blood-cell adhesion. Meaningful data of this type has been infrequently published on candidate hydrogel coatings. To understand the structure and function of the coatings, it is also necessary to have data on water adsorption, interpenetration with substrata, chemical composition, especially if an energetic reaction is used in the preparation, crosslinking, and gel fraction. Techniques for determining all these properties reliably on coatings a few microns thick have not been worked out in general, although some results have been reported. Considerable effort has been expended by some groups on determination of water uptake, using direct weighing, hydrophilic dyes, or Fisher titration.

The methods which have been used to prepare hydrogel coatings on organic polymer substrata have been simple casting and adhesion, formation of interpenetrating networks, chemical grafting initiated by ceric ion from solutions of hydrogel monomer onto the substratum, ultraviolet light, ionizing radiation, and activation of monomer vapor with atomic hydrogen or ozone. This review will attempt to cover these methods insofar as the products have been characterized and described in the open literature. The more unique of the investigations published only in government reports will also be cited.

HYDROGEN COATINGS APPLIED BY SIMPLE ADHESION

The earliest attempt to use hydrogel in contact with blood appears to be with charcoal coated with HEMA (2-hydroxyethylmethacrylate) in a hemoperfusion apparatus [3]. The particles were prepared by polymerizing 10% ethanolic HEMA solution in the presence of an equal mass of activated carbon, drying the product at 95°C, and reconstituting it with saline. The dry product contained either 4% or 2% pHEMA. Physical characterization was not complete with these materials, but biological performance was favorable according to all the cited investigations: only 20% removal of platelets, returning to normal in 24 hours, no blood clots, no carbon emboli found in tissue, recovery of patients poisoned by barbiturate or glutethemide, and efficient removal from blood of paracetamol, ethanol, acetyl salicylate, and others.

Although it is possible to spread hydrophilic solutions on flat plastic surfaces if the surfaces are made compatible by treatment with an oxidizing agent [4], adhesion is usually poor and most investigators have turned to other methods.

INTERPENETRATING NETWORKS

A hydrogel film can be firmly anchored to a hydrophobic substratum if the two polymeric networks mutually interpenetrate. A practical application has been reported for hemodialysis membranes of cellulose or collodion made hemocompatible with coatings of polyvinylpyrrolidone, pAAm (polyacrylamide), or pHEMA [5]. The hydrogels were not well characterized, but the coatings lowered the permeability to phosphate by an order of magnitude. This appears to be a result of the high degree of crosslinking necessary for a mechanically stable gel; the permeability of lightly crosslinked pAAm, which was too fragile to serve as a practical coating, was satisfactory.

Preparation of the above system was facilitated by the similarly of the surface energies of the coating and substratum. A hydrogel composite with polyvinylchloride can also be formed by hot-pressing films of the components. For example, HEMA was copolymerized with lauryl methacrylate in methanol to prepare a thermoplastic hydrophilic polymer. This was heated and spread into a 1-mm thick film in contact with a sheet of polyvinylchloride and hot-pressed. These sheets could be fabricated into hydrogel-coated equipment for extracorporeal circulation. The lining would form a hydrogel when equilibrated with water [6], which was described as compatible with blood.

Interpenetrating networks can also be prepared by polymerizing the hydrogel *in situ* in the substratum, the monomer being introduced either dissolved in a penetrating solvent or from the vapor. Kronick has described an interpenetrating network of polyacrylamide on polyetherurethane [7]. The monomer was introduced in a 50% solution in glycol-methoxyethanol onto a substratum of polyetherurethane block copolymer which it penetrated. After the volatile methoxyethanol evaporated, the polymerization was initiated with atomic hydrogen by a process to be described below. Although inextricable interpenetrating networks which absorb water are formed by this technique or by introducing the monomer from the vapor, it appeared that the interpenetrating network extended to the surface, with no discrete hydrogel coating. The water uptake of this network was determined to be only 14%. This material was tested for blood compatibility by the spinning-disk method of Leonard [8]. A sample of the grafted polyetherurethane formed the face of a disk spinning at 400 RPM in blood from a cannulated dog. Values of plasma protein found deposited on the surface after 4 minutes compared to untreated polyetherurethane (sample/polyetherurethane) were albumin, 0.36/0.47, gamma globulin 0.61/1.38, and fibrinogen 0.90/2.48, respectively. Even with relatively low water content, the treated surfaces were more inert to plasma proteins than the control. Both the albumin and gamma globulin increased during the test period: the fibrinogen remained the same.

CHEMICAL GRAFTING WITH OXIDIZING AGENTS

A very interesting method of covalently grafting hydrogels to certain polymeric substrata from aqueous solution has been described by Halpern [9]. The substrate surface is placed in contact with a solution of acrylamide, optional crosslinker, and ceric nitrate. For example, a sample of polyetherurethane block copolymer was immersed in 1.4 M acrylamide and 7.5×10^{-3} M ceric ammonium nitrate at 25°C for 15 min. The products applied to films of two types of polyetherurethanes were examined by several methods. Cross sections were dyed with methylene blue and observed in an optical microscope. Only a superficial layer from 2 to 10 microns thick, depending upon preparation conditions, was seen to be dyed. The thickness of the coatings after drying could also be measured, giving the degree of swelling. Although this important quantity was in the range found gravimetrically, the two types of measurement did not agree on the same samples from a series of preparations. The critical surface tension was found to vary from 25 to 31.5 dyne/cm, implying hydrophobicity, although it was similar to values reported for some biological surfaces.

The tenacity was not affected by the coating treatment, but, on drying, the flexural deformation under a standard stress increased in the treated film above the value for the untreated; there was no effect in hydrated samples. It was observed that appreciable surface erosion took place under the prolonged shear stress of flowing water. These changes were observed by scanning electron microscopy, which revealed what resembled eroded lakes and islands of remaining hydrogel in coatings which had been prepared without crosslinker. The changes were much less marked when 0.4% methylene bisacrylamide had been included in the polymerizate.

The possibility that an interpenetrating network is formed at the surface must be considered in this system. The infrared spectrum determined by multiple internal reflectance of a coating on the polyetherurethane with composition 3(1000/425)(70/30)1X shows only features of pAAm or of pHEMA, depending on the monomer used. However, the properties of pAAm coatings depend on the particular polyetherurethane substratum. If a "softer" polymer is coated, thicker films which swell more in water are obtained than on the "hard" material cited above. No demarkation between surface grafted layer and substratum is observed in SEM cross sections of this coated material. Further, extraction of monomer after the coating treatment on either material requires about 72 hours, and it has been determined that, in both cases, most of the AAm extracted comes from the bulk substratum. Therefore, the possibility of interpenetration always exists in this type of system, the extent depending on the particular substratum.

A number of variations of these preparations have been tested *in vivo* and *ex vivo* [9]. The *ex vivo* tests have been the more consistent, showing the surfaces to be most inert in interaction with dog-blood platelets, but not completely inert. Typical results from the Leonard spinning-disk adhesion test [8] conducted for 4 min were (pAAM/polyetherurethane): gamma globulin (0.4/1.5 μg/cm^2), fibrinogen (0.8/2.2μg/cm^2), and platelets (0.05/11.0 cells/900μ^2). Steady-state adhesion was reached in 0.3 min for gamma globulin, 1 min for fibrinogen, and 0.5 min for platelets. The results for proteins were obtained on pure solutions; from platelets, *ex vitro* with dog's blood. The advantages of the coating for hemostasis were less marked, however, in *in-vivo* tests. Five small rings coated with polyetherurethane and pAAm, implanted in the renal artery of dogs in the Kusserow renal-embolus test [10], all showed some thrombotic material. Two had only thin coatings after three days, while three were partially occluded. All the specimens caused renal infarcts; since these occur downstream from the implanted test ring, they indicate that material embolized from the implantation site (probably from the surface of the test ring) and became lodged in the kidney.

Test rings similarly coated for the Gott vena-cava test [11] were also tested for thrombogenesis. Like the tests for renal emboli, these were too few to be statistically significant characterizations of any one method of preparation of the pAAm coating. For any one method, about one half of the tested samples (about 2-3) would have small thrombi after a 2-week implantation, while the other half would result in early death of the test dog or complete occlusion of the vena cava.

The discrepancy between *in-vivo* and *in-vitro* results must be accepted as state-of-the-art in testing blood compatibility. Besides the question of relevancy of particular tests, consideration must be given to differences in handling the specimens, changes in the surface, etc. For example, the specimens in some cases were shipped across thousands of miles in unsterile water from the site of sample preparation to that of testing. Also, the flat film samples used in the *in-vitro* and *ex-vivo* tests could be prepared with greater control and perfection than the cylinders used in the *in-vivo* tests.

ACTIVE-VAPOR METHODS

Devices for vascular applications are fabricated with extraordinary care from medical-grade polymers, which should be of the highest purity. Immersion of such items in liquids for the purpose of coating them exposes them to the risk of imbibing dissolved impurities, which might be difficult to remove later. Vapor-coating methods meet this drawback, since impurities are all volatile and present in a very dilute form. Another advantage of vapor coating is that complex shapes can be treated with rapid penetration of reagents into crevices without local stirring (Fib. 1B). The slight volatility of HEMA permits it to be deposited onto plastic surfaces from its vapor at reduced pressure. Yamauchi describes such a method, in which polyvinyl chloride is first activated with a mixture of 1.4% ozone in oxygen. HEMA is then deposited on the surface from the vapor and polymerized by heating at 98°C at 5 torr [12]. A concomitant increase in thromboresistance was reported.

Oxygen and ozone probably activate polymeric surfaces by forming reactive oxides or peroxides. Such reactions lead to degradation and oily products. Atomic hydrogen, on the other hand, results largely in hydrogen abstraction, leading to metastable free radicals and internal crosslinks. Although degradation proceeds as well as crosslinking, in all polymer substrates examined so far (polymeric hydrocarbons, silicones, polyetherurethanes, polyesters, polystyrene, and others) the net change was an increase in network formation [13]. The lifetimes of the free radicals are distributed over a range from seconds to days, and so can be used to initiate grafted polymer chains if a monomer is introduced to them shortly after they are formed.

The vapor of atomic hydrogen is extremely reactive, forming free radicals in solid polymers to a depth of approximately 10^{-5} cm. Ingalls et al. [14], treating finely divided polystyrene with atomic hydrogen, formed an average radical concentration of 10^{-3} M with lifetimes of about 2 hr at room temperature. Results from radiation grafting show that this is fully adequate to initiate grafting polymerization reactions with large yields. The active vapors are stable enough to be conducted several feet along internal surfaces to be treated, which are located remote from the vapor-activating apparatus. Thus the choice of this apparatus can be arbitrary: a microwave discharge, an electric arc, or simply a heated filament. In the equipment which we use, a 1:1 mixture of hydrogen and helium at 3 torr flows through an intense electrical discharge in a 100-W microwave cavity, where some of the hydrogen is dissociated into its atoms. It flows into a chamber where the sample to be treated is located, at which point it is 3% dissociated, giving a vapor with 10^{-8} M atomic hydrogen.

A diagram of our apparatus appears in Figure 2. Hydrogen and helium at atmospheric pressure, flowing at 100 ml/min and 75 ml/min, respectively, are mixed and introduced into the vacuum flow system at 2 torr. The mixture passes through a microwave cavity and is excited with 100W/cm³ of microwave power at 2450 MHz. Monomer, in the form of vapor, is introduced into the reactor by distillation from the heated reservoir. The mixture in the reservoir comprises 1.5 g acrylamde, 80 mg ethylene glycol dimethacrylate, 3 g glycerol, and 0.1 g CuCl. A magnetically actuated valve located below the active-vapor inlet allows interruption of the flow of monomer vapor. The sample to be treated is

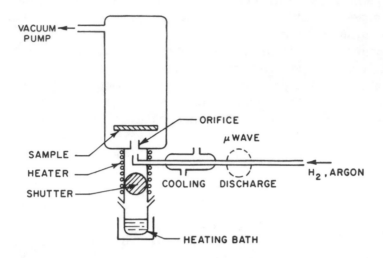

Figure 2. Apparatus for vapor-phase grafting acrylate hydrogels to surfaces by means of atomic-hydrogen initiated polymerization.

mounted 3 cm from the orifice inside the reactor chamber. With no heat supplied to the reservoir and with the monomer port closed, active vapor impinges on the surface to be treated for 3 min. The reservoir is then heated to 95°C, and the monomer port is opened for 1 sec. At this point, after the monomer port is closed the hydrogen concentration in the active vapor is reduced to 10% for 10 sec. The monomer port is then intermittently opened for 1-sec intervals and held closed for 10-sec intervals to build up layers of polyacrylamide on the surface.

Polyacrylamide without crosslinker was prepared on a cold finger at the sample position of the reactor. The product was collected as a solution in ethylene glycol on the end of the glass cold finger. The molecular weights of soluble polyacrylamide were calculated from the inherent viscosity determined at 25°, using the Mark-Houwink equation [6]:

$$[\eta] = 6.80 \times 10^{-4} M_n^{-0.66}. \tag{1}$$

The molecular weights of polyacrylamide samples polymerized with different concentrations of atomic hydrogen in the vapor are listed in Table 1.

In a free-radical system which is polymerizing without chain transfer, every molecule continues to grow until it is terminated by combining

Table 1. Viscometric Determination of Molecular Weight of Active-Hydrogen Polymerized Polyacrylamide.

Relative Active Hydrogen	Inherent Viscosity	$\overline{M}_n$
1	1.3	95,000
3	1.04	66,000
4	0.43	18,000
5	0.54	25,000
6	0.78	43,000
7	0.39	14,000

with another growing molecule. According to Flory's theory of free-radical polymerization, the degree of polymerization is then given by:

$$\textbf{Constant} \times [H°]^{-1/2} \tag{2}$$

in which $[H°]$ is the atomic-hydrogen concentration in the condensed phase. The molecular weight therefore decreases with increasing concentrations of active hydrogen. This is in agreement with the data in Table 1. We have estimated by calorimetry of the recombining atoms that the concentration of the atomic hydrogen is about 2.8×10^{-8}M in the vapor. It is not known how this correlates with the concentration in the condensed phase, which, from the low molecular weight of the product, appears to be higher than usual for the conventional polymerization system, which yields typical values of molecular weight of over 10^6 Dalton.

This treatment was used to modify several different materials with pHEMA or with pAAm. By use of electron-probe analysis the water content, thickness and surface topography of the coatings could be examined *in situ*. To carry out this analysis, a series of conventional pAAm samples were polymerized with different amounts of crosslinker, to vary the degree of water uptake in the series. The samples were equilibrated with aqueous solutions of a low molecular-weight solute which contained a heavy atom. For example, solutions 0.1M in KCl, KBr, or $AgNO_3$

were used. The samples were lyophilized, fractured, and examined with a scanning electron microscope in its energy-dispersed X-ray mode. The X-ray fluorescence characteristic of the heavy atom was counted and was calibrated against the amount of water imbibed by the sample at equilibrium, measured gravimetrically. Water contents were varied over the range 50 to 90 percent. To study an unknown sample, it was soaked in one of the above solutions, lyophilized, and fractured. The fracture surface was examined by scanning electron microscopy and also in the energy-dispersed X-ray mode, as above. The X-ray emission was compared to the calibration curve obtained with the conventional samples to determine the amount of aqueous solution imbibed. The method is internally compensated for partition of the solute between the aqueous and gel phases and the collapse of the gel during drying, which would increase the local concentration of fluorescent solute. The method is the more sensitive the heavier the atom, silver emitting more X-rays than potassium.

A sample of polypropylene coated with pAAm by the atomic-hydrogen method described above is shown in cross section in Figure 3. The white areas in the SEM of Figure 3A are shown to be hydrogel in the silver map of Figure 3B. The hydrophilic region is sharply defined.

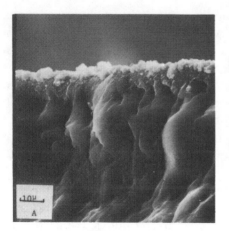

Figure 3. Cross section of polypropylene coated with pAAm from the vapor by the active-hydrogen grafting technique described in the text, using the apparatus of Figure 2. A. Scanning electron micrograph. B. Silver-ion penetration map of the same field as A.

Besides preparing indicator maps, the electron-probe analyzer can also scan the cross-section and produce a quantitative profile of indicator concentration. An interesting example of this is shown in Figure 3 for a sample of polyetherurethane block copolymer vapor-coated with pAAm by the atomic-hydrogen method. The silver-ion X-ray fluorescence of a sample of conventional pAAm which imbibed 50 percent water is shown on the left, the height of the trace being proportional to silver concentration in the gel. This trace was stored in the memory of the minicomputer attached to the analyzer, while that on the right was being accumulated for the profile of silver ion across the cross section of the coated sample. Although the surface hydrogel contains more than 50 percent water, the modification is not limited to a superficial layer. The grafting treatment has formed what is apparently an interpenetrating network of pAAm and polyetherurethane extending several hundred microns into the substratum. Bulk properties of the sample were thereby altered. The vapor method, therefore, is unsuitable for surface grafting onto polyetherurethane, because of a high affinity of AAm for the polymer.

The penetration of AAm from aqueous solution is much less than from the vapor because water, in which it is very soluble, lowers its activity even at a concentration of several molar. If the interfacial tension between this monomer solution and polyetherurethane is lowered by the addition of a detergent or ethanol, a thin film can be spread on the hydrophobic substratum and subsequently polymerized with atomic hydrogen. In this case the hydrophilic layer, 80μm thick, is confined to the surface according to the silver-ion profile, but the silver concentration in the superficial layer indicates a water content of only 15 or 20%. This low water content is probably due to interdiffusion of components between the substratum and pAAm.

GRAFTING WITH NON-IONIZING RADIATION

Photosensitized grafting has been described by Oster for modifying the surface of polyethylene, polyethylene terephthalate, polyacrylonitrile, nylon, natural rubber, and cellulose with pAAm, polyvinylpyrrolidone, and polyoctylacrylamide [15]. A photosensitizer such as benzophenone is diffused into the surface of the substratum, which is then illuminated with near ultraviolet light in the presence of an aqueous solution of the monomer. These products are unsuitable for medical applications because the slightly soluble photosensitizer would slowly leach from the surface in use. Kronick has used the method, however, to build up thick films of pAAm onto less swellable substrata such as cellulose by using ferric ion as the photosensitizer [16]. The method is also advantageous in building up thicker films of pAAm onto the thin coatings obtained by the active-hydrogen method. An SEM and a silver-penetration map showing a coating with greater than 50% water content are shown in Figure 4 for a sample of polypropylene which has been coated with pAAm by the active-hydrogen vapor method; then impregnated with saturated ferric chloride solution (pH 2.0), drained, immersed in the monomer solution, and illuminated immediately with ultraviolet light for two minutes. No penetrating reagents were used, although immersion in any liquid reagent has the drawbacks mentioned earlier.

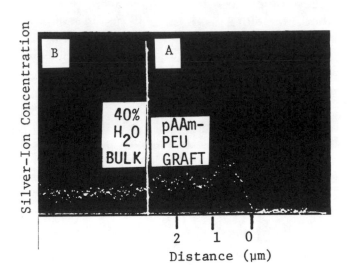

Figure 4. Silver-ion penetration profile across a polyetherurethane film sample which had been treated by the pAAm vapor-phase grafting technique with atomic hydrogen (A), compared with the silver-ion level in a piece of pAAm which had been polymerized from aqueous solution by a conventional free-radical method (B).

Samples prepared in this way showed the same discrepant behavior between *in-vivo* and *ex-vivo* tests with blood as did the chemical oxidation-grated materials of Halpern, et al. Four-minute tests for platelet adhesion in the spinning-disk apparatus of Leonard [8] gave, for two samples, 4.0 and 0.4 cells per $900\mu^2$, compared to 17.0 cells/$900\mu^2$ for untreated polyetherurethane.

Determinations were also made on adsorption of proteins from single-protein solutions. In these experiments, carried out in the laboratories of Dr. Leo Vroman [17], the disks were immersed in normal human plasma, and the adsorbed proteins were measured either immunologically or by their ability to correct the clotting behavior of human blood deficient in one or another clotting factor. Tests were run for fibrinogen adsorption, fibrinogen "conversion," and adsorption of Factors XI and XII and 7-S γ-globulin. Some Factor XII was adsorbed, correcting deficient plasma by 7.8%; adsorbed Factor XI corrected by 37.9%. A single sample showed no adsorption of any of these proteins; this sample had the thickest polyacrylamide coating.

Although fibrinogen and gamma globulins deposit onto many surfaces within 1 sec. the pAAm-grafted material showed no immunochemical evidence of the protein after 5 sec., but it did appear after 10 min. in a platelet-adhesive ("unconverted") form.

RADIATION GRAFTING

Although radiation grafting would appear to be a general method for coating implants with hydrogel [18], its feasibility depends on the radiation chemistry of the system. In principle the radiation should form free radicals in the substratum polymer, which add to the monomer and initiate the polymerization. If both reagents are present, the value of G(radicals) for substratum polymer must be much greater than that for the monomer, or the main product will be hydrogel homopolymer rather than graft copolymer. The analysis is complicated by the desired structure for the product, which should have a graft copolymer at the interface between the unmodified substratum and a hydrogel homopolymer coating: formation of homopolymer near the interface is therefore actually desirable.

In the earliest report of the method used for medical purposes, silicone rubber was coated with polyvinyl pyrrolidone [19]. The surface coating could be visualized and measured by eosin staining, sectioning, and microscopy. The rubber swells about 2% in the monomer, causing interpenetration of the two networks when only small amounts of water were used (20%). Water also accelerated the polymerization of the graft. Grafts about 125μm thick were obtained, containing about 50% water in the grafted layers considered as homogeneous polyvinylpyrrolidone.

The products from the radiation-grafting technique have been examined extensively for silicone rubber as a substratum by Hoffman and coworkers. The data, which included gravimetry, water absorption isotherms, scanning electron micrographs, wetting angles, and infrared spectra, indicate that superficial layers of polymer were readily obtained with water contents which resembled those from typical solution polymerized pHEMA, poly(propylene glycol monoacrylate), pAAm, poly(N-methylacrylamide), polymethacrylic acid, and their copolymers with vinyl pyrrolidone. Homopolymerization was suppressed by addition of Cu^{++} to the monomer. Considerable interpenetration was observed by attenuated total-reflectance IR studies between silicone rubber and poly(HEMA/vinyl pyrrolidone) [20]. The results of these investigations are extensively reviewed elsewhere in this volume.

ACKNOWLEDGEMENT

For the photograph in Figure 1B and early realization of the vapor-phase method of atomic-hydrogen initiated grafting, we acknowledge the contributions of Dr. Harvey Scott.

REFERENCES

1. Andrade, J.D. Interfacial Phenomena and Biomaterials. Medical Instrumentation 7:110 (1973).
2. Wichterle, O., and Lim, D. Hydrophilic Gels for Biological Use. Nature 185:117 (1960).
3. Andrade, J.D. Trans. Amer. Soc. Artif. Int. Organs 17:222 (1971).
4. Lundell, E.O., Kwiatkowski, G.T., Byck, J.S., Osterholtz, F.D., Creasy, W.S., and Stewart, D.D. Biological and Physical Characteristics of Some Polyelectrolytes in Hydrogels for Medical and Related Applications. J.D. Andrade, ed., A.C.S. Symposium Series No. 31, Washington, American Chemical Society, pp. 305-328 (1976).
5. Moise, O., Sideman, S., Hoffer, E., Rousseau, I., and Better, O.S. Membrane Permeability for Inorganic Phosphate Ion. J. Biomed. Mater. Res. 11:903-913 (1977).
6. Makashima, T., Yamauchi, K., and Takakura, K. Blood- and Transfusion Fluid-Compatible Poly(Vinyl Chloride) Equipment. Japan Kokai Patent No. 77-22070 02/19/77.

7. Kronick, P. Active-Vapor Grafted Hydrogels. Polymer Preprints 16(2):441-445 (1975).
8. Kochwa, S., Litwak, R.S., Rosenfield, R.E., and Leonard, E.F. Blood Elements at Foreign Surfaces: In Vitro Evaluation of Biomaterials in a Spinning Disk Apparatus. Ann. N.Y. Acad. Sci. 283:457-472 (1977).
9. Halpern, B.D., Solomon, O., and Chowhan, D.G. Polymer Studies Related to Prosthetic Cardiac Materials which are Non-Clotting at a Blood Interface. Contract No. NO1-HV-6-1124. National Heart and Lung Institute, National Institutes of Health, Bethesda, Md. Annual Report June 1976. PB 255 913/AS.
10. Kusserow, B. The Use of Pathologic Techniques in the Evaluation of Emboli from Prosthetic Devices. Bull. N.Y. Acad. Med. 48:468 (1972).
11. Gott, V.L. Heparin Bonding on Colloidal Graphite Surfaces. Science 142:297 (1963).
12. Yamauchi, J. Anticoagulative Tubings. Japan Kokai Patent No. 75-38790 4/10/75.
13. Hansen, R.H., and Schonhorn, H. A New Technique for Preparing Low Surface Energy Polymers for Adhesive Bonding. Polymer Lett. 4:203-209 (1966).
14. Ingalls, R.B. and Ward, I.A. Electron Spin Resonance Spectra of Free-Radical Intermediates Formed by Reaction of Polystyrene with Atoms of Hydrogen and Deuterium. J. Chem. Phys. 35:370-1 (1961).
15. Oster, G., Brit. Patent 856,884, Dec. 21, 1960.
16. Kronick, P.L. Fabrication and Characterization of Grafted Hydrogel Coatings Prepared by Active-Hydrogen Techhniques for Heart-Assist Devices. Contract No. NO1-HV-1-2017. National Heart and Lung Institute, National Institutes of Health, Bethesda, Md. Annual Report Jan. 1977. PB 264-748.
17. Vroman, L., Adams, A.L., Klings, M., Fischer, G.C., Munoz, P.C., and Solensky, R.P. Reactions of Formed Elements of Blood with Plasma Proteins at Interfaces. Ann. N.Y. Acad. Sci. 283:65-76 (1977).
18. Chapiro, A. "Radiation Chemistry of Polymer Systems." Interscience, New York, 1962.
19. Yasuda, H., and Refojo, M.F. Graft Copolymerization of Vinylpyrrolidone onto Polymethylsiloxane. J. Polymer Sci. A 2:5093-8 (1964).
20. Ratner, B.D., and Hoffman, A.S. The Effect of Cupric Ion on the Radiation Grafting and N-Vinyl-2-Pyrrolidone and other Hydrophilic Monomers onto Silicone Rubber." J. Appl. Polymer Sci. 18:3183-3204 (1974).

OPHTHALMIC HYDROGELS*

Miguel F. Refojo, D.Sc.

*Eye Research Institute of Retina Foundation
and Department of Ophthalmology
Harvard Medical School
Boston, Mass.*

ABSTRACT

Hydrogels are polymers that swell to equilibrium in aqueous media. Natural and synthetic hydrogels have been used in ophthalmology because they physically resemble the tissues of the eye. The most important application of hydrogels in ophthalmology is for the manufacture of soft corneal contact lenses. The experimental applications of hydrogels in eye surgery — artificial corneas, drainage devices for relief of intraocular pressure in glaucoma, artificial intraocular lenses, vitreous implants, and scleral buckling materials in retinal detachment surgery — are reviewed.

KEY WORDS

Hydrogels, Hydrophilic polymers, Contact lenses, Keratoprosthesis, Intraocular lenses, Glaucoma drainage devices, Vitreous substitutes, Scleral buckling for retinal detachment surgery, Materials in the eye, Ocular implants.

*Supported by USPHS grant EY-00327 from the National Eye Institute, National Institutes of Health

Hydrogels are coherent systems rich in water; they are made up of two principal components: a constant solid component consisting of a polymer network, and a variable liquid component, either water or an aqueous solution. The aqueous component can undergo exchange with the environment by diffusion or evaporation. Permanent hydrogels are covalently cross-linked and are insoluble. Reversible hydrogels may be dissolved when certain solutes are added to the aqueous component, or, if they are thermal hydrogels, the gel may be liquefied by changes in temperature.

Essentially, hydrogels are a type of gel in which the polymer network is hydrophilic and the liquid component is aqueous. Gels can be made by cross-linking already-formed polymers, or by simultaneously polymerizing and cross-linking various monomers. Gels obtained from the copolymerization of monomers containing a relatively small amount of a cross-linking agent were studied as early as 1936 by Staudinger, who found that the amount of liquid that is bound when a gel swells is inversely proportional to the extent of cross-linking in the polymer network.

Hydrogels obtained from natural products, such as gelatin and agar, have been in existence for many years. Since 1949, gelatin has been used as an absorbable implant material in general surgery; it was first used in retina surgery in 1954, and in glaucoma surgery in 1958. Currently, the principal use of gelatin in ophthalmology is as scleral implants for retinal detachment surgery when a temporary indentation of the sclera is desired [1].

A hydrogel formed by cross-linking poly(vinyl alcohol) with formaldehyde was among the first materials used as surgical implants, particularly in the form of soft sponges. It has long been known that aqueous solutions of poly(vinyl alcohol) containing small amounts of certain azo dyes of the Congo red type yield highly rigid gells on cooling. Such hydrogels vary in rigidity, depending on dye and polymer concentration, and on molecular weight and degree of acetate substitution in the poly(vinyl alcohol). The gel formation is thermal and reversible. Custodis introduced Polyviol as an implant for scleral buckling in retinal detachment surgery. This gel consists of poly(vinyl alcohol) mixed with sufficient Congo red to yield the desired solidity and elasticity. Custodis found that postoperative complications such as extrusion of the implant or infection were rare. However, when Schepens et al. [2] used the Custodis procedure, they found a high rate of complications, which included irritation of the orbital tissues and relatively frequent infections around the implant, but concluded that the softness and elasticity of the poly(vinyl alcohol) implant were desirable qualities. Poly(vinyl alcohol) is no longer used in ophthalmology, and the Custodis technique for the treatment of retinal detachment is performed most often with silicone sponge implants.

Acrylamide hydrogels, commonly used in biochemistry laboratories for gel electrophoresis, were first described in 1959 as strong, flexible, transparent hydrogels obtained by simultaneous polymerization and crosslinking of acrylamide and N',N-methylene bis-acrylamide [3]. Acrylamide hydrogels have been used experimentally as vitreous implants, but have not proven to be clinically useful. Similar to acrylamide hydrogels are the hydroxyalkyl (or glycol) acrylate hydrogels first described in 1960 by Wichterle and Lim, who proposed these materials for possible use as surgical implants [4]. Hydrogels of a glycol monomethacrylate crosslinked with a glycol dimethacrylate offered the following advantages: they could be made to contain different amounts of water at equilibrium swelling, were relatively resistant to hydrolysis and easy to sterilize, and were apparently well tolerated when implanted in experimental animals. Among the properties that made hydrogels desirable for biomedical use were their softness, their permeability to electrolytes and, presumably, to some metabolites, and their general physical resemblance to living human tissues, with respect to water content.

In the early sixties, the field of biomaterials was not very advanced and surgeons often used commercial plastics as surgical implants, with little or no knowledge of their purity or composition. The fact that hydrogels consist of an open and relatively porous network structure added to their advantages for use as biomaterials because prolonged washing in water would rid the implant of impurities. Residual catalyst and monomers and any other diffusible impurities can be washed out of hydrogels, leaving an essentially pure polymer. The transparency of most acrylic hydrogels led Wichterle and Lim to recognize that their potential would best be realized in the field of ophthalmology. However, acrylic hydrogels have been used at least experimentally at one time or another in almost all medical specialties [5].

Of all possible uses of hydrogels in biomedicine, contact lenses are the single most important application. The use of hydrogels in several surgical procedures has also been investigated. This chapter will deal only with those uses pertaining to ophthalmology.

Synthetic materials have been widely used in the eye: for artificial corneas, crystalline lens, drainage tubes for release of intraocular fluids in glaucoma surgery, as vitreous implants, and in scleral buckling procedures for retinal detachment surgery [6]. Some of these uses, such as implantation of artificial corneas, and drainage tubes in glaucoma surgery, are relatively rare, and are done only in very specific cases by a limited number of ophthalmic surgeons. However, the implantation of intraocular artificial lenses has become a fairly common operation, but is often restricted to certain categories of patients. Scleral buckling with an artificial implant material is currently a widely used procedure for the treatment of retinal detachment.

Corneal Contact Lenses

Of particular interest for their economic as well as social significance are contact lenses. Although contact lenses are not surgically implanted devices, they are used in very close contact with the eye, and their physiological performance depends greatly on the material used to make the lens. Contact lenses are optical devices, usually made of a synthetic polymer, that are placed over the cornea of the eye and remain between the lids and the cornea when the eye blinks. The main purpose of contact lenses is vision correction, but certain types of lenses are often used medically to treat corneal diseases or to protect the cornea in patients with certain eye problems. In the latter cases, the contact lenses are called therapeutic or bandage lenses. A further use of hydrogel contact lenses, which takes advantage of their absorbing properties, is for prolonged delivery of drugs to the eye [7].

Corneal contact lenses must provide the optical correction required by the patient without compromising the integrity of the eye tissues. The fit of the lens on the cornea has to be such that any chance of mechanical irritation is minimized. Equally important is the requirement that the corneal physiology under the lens remain as close as possible to its normal state. The corneal surface must always be wet and oxygenated. This wetness is normally provided by the tear film. With a well-fit hard contact lens, tears are usually pumped under the lens by blinking. With a hydrophilic lens, which is in much closer contact to the corneal surface than the hard lens, tear pumping may not be as important and the lens itself may provide the wetness required by the corneal surface.

The cornea is an avascular tissue that metabolically maintains its thickness and transparency by consuming oxygen. Normally, oxygena-

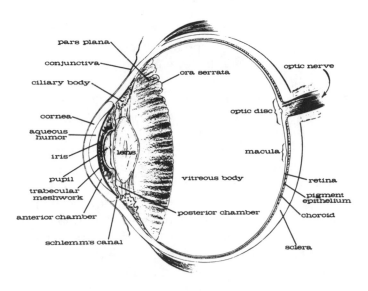

Figure 1. Schematic representation of the eye.

tion of the corneal surface takes place through the tear film that supplies the cornea with oxygen from the air. When the eyelids are closed, as during sleep, oxygenation is supplied to the corneal surface from the blood capillary vessels of the palpebral conjunctiva which comprises the posterior part of the eyelids. When the corneal surface is deprived of oxygen below a minimum requirement of about 15 mm Hg partial pressure, the cornea swells and becomes hazy. Thus, a contact lens must not disrupt the oxygenation of the cornea under it, although it may decrease the available oxygen to a certain tolerable level. Oxygenation of the cornea under a contact lens is achieved by exchange of oxygenated tears under the lens (activated by blinking), by oxygen transport through the lens, or by a combination of both.

The contact lens field was reviewed recently from a materials point of view by this author [8]. Different types of contact lenses are currently available, including the so-called hard poly(methyl methacrylate) contact lenses, and some newer hard lenses with improved oxygen permeability such as those made from cellulose acetate butyrate. Flexible contact lenses with excellent oxygen permeability are made from silicone rubber. Silicone rubber is very lipophilic, and even after various treatments to render the surface of silicone lenses hydrophilic, these lenses have been plagued with difficulties, particularly due to lipid contamination and decreased wettability leading to intolerance.

The original hydrophilic soft, or hydrogel, contact lenses introduced by Wichterle and Lim were made of 2-hydroxyethyl methacrylate cross-linked with ethylene glycol dimethacrylate. Lenses of this composition are currently made under the trade names of Soflens (polymacon) (Bausch & Lomb) and Hydron (National Patent Development Corp.). (The capitalized trade name of a lens is sometimes followed by a non-proprietary name in parentheses, which is the name given by the United States Adopted Names Council.)

For a given thickness of hydrogel contact lens, oxygen permeability increases with increased water content. High oxygen permeability in a durable hydrogel lens is a desirable objective which can be achieved by making ultrathin lenses of lower hydration or by making less thin lenses of higher hydration. Of course, an ultrathin high-water-content lens would be ideal, but higher-water-content materials are in general more fragile, and are more durable when they are thicker. Furthermore, because hydrogel lenses are cut in the dry state during fabrication, the thickness of a finished hydrogel lens is limited by the thickness at which the lens can be cut when dry. Thus, if, for example, the minimum thickness at which a lens can be cut when dry is about 0.05 mm thick, then its thickness increases at equilibrium in water by about 18% to 0.059 mm thick if the equilibrium hydration of the lens is 40% water; its thickness will increase by 45% to about 0.072 mm if the equilibrium hydration of the lens is 80% water.

A centrifugal casting method for making hydrogel lenses has been developed by Wichterle. In this technique a prepolymer solution is polymerized in a mold rotating about its central axis. In these spun-cast lenses the optical power depends on the concave surface curvature of the lens that is obtained by the spinning of the mold during the casting process. The spin-casting procedure of fabrication of hydrogel contact lenses is currently used only by Bausch & Lomb to manufacture Soflens contact lenses.

The most widely used procedure for the manufacture of hydrogel contact lenses is the more or less standardized technique of lathe-cutting that is similar to the original technique used to manufacture hard poly(methyl methacrylate) lenses. The polymer is usually produced in the dry state by bulk polymerization of the prepolymer mixture in molds that yield semifinished lenses, or in the form of rods which are then cut into blanks. Some manufacturers obtain the polymer in the swollen state, presumably to diminish bubble formation during polymerization and to avoid polymer internal stresses commonly found in bulk-polymerized rods. The swollen polymer is thoroughly washed in water, and is then allowed to dry under controlled conditions to obtain the hard plastic (xerogel) ready for lathing.

Transparent hydrogels of 2-hydroxyethyl methacrylate polymer contain a maximum of about 40% water at equilibrium swelling. Higher-water-content hydrogels of the polymer can be made, but they are hazy to opaque. Copolymers of 2-hydroxyethyl methacrylate with some other more hydrophilic monomers produce hydrogels with higher levels of hydration. Thus, Wichterle and Lim copolymerized 2-hydroxyethyl methacrylate with some of the homologous esters of glycol monomethacrylate, such as di-, tri-, and tetraethylene glycol monomethacrylates, adding some glycol dimethacrylate as a cross-linking agent, to obtain higher-water-content hydrogels.

Vinylpyrrolidone copolymerized with 2-hydroxyethyl methacrylate is used to produce several types of hydrogel contact lenses, such as the Naturvue (hefilcon A) lens of Milton Roy Soft Contact Lens Inc. Graft or block copolymers of 2-hydroxyethyl methacrylate onto poly(vinylpyrrolidone) are used in another type of hydrogel lens, the Softcon (vifilcon A) lens of American Optical Corp.

Another approach to the problem of producing high-water-content hydrogels with improved mechanical properties has been by means of copolymers of one or several hydrophilic monomers with one or several hydrophobic monomers, with a standard cross-linking agent, usually a glycol dimethacrylate or other divinyl monomer. A commonly used hydrophobic monomer is methyl methacrylate, which is copolymerized with vinylpyrrolidone to obtain Sauflon (lidofilcon) contact lenses of Sauflon International, Inc. Hydroxyethyl methacrylate copolymerized with methacrylic acid and vinylpyrrolidone is used in the Permalens (perfilcon A) contact lenses of Cooper Laboratories, Inc. Hydroxyethyl methacrylate, with methyl methacrylate and vinylpyrrolidone, and divinyl benzene as cross-linking agent, is used in the Aquaflex (tetrafilcon A) of UCO Optics, Inc., and in the Aosoft lens of American Optical Corp. Poly(hydroxyethyl methacrylate-co-sodium methacrylate-co-2-ethyl-2-(hydroxymethyl)-1, 3-propanediol trimethacrylate) is the hydrogel used in Hydro-Marc (etafilcon A) of Frontier Contact Lens, Inc. Poly(hydroxyethyl methacrylate-co-methacrylic acid-co-ethylene dimethacrylate) is used in Tresoft (ocufilcon A) of Urocon International. A copolymer of hydroxyethyl methacrylate with an acrylic derivative,

N-(1,1-dimethyl-3-oxobutyl)acrylamide (also known as diacetone acrylamide), cross-linked with 1,3-propanediol trimethacrylate, forms the hydrogel of HydroCurve II (bufilcon A) contact lenses of Soft Lenses, Inc.

Usually, high-water-content hydrogel contact lenses have the problems of fragility, poor reproducibility, and, because of the looser network structure, susceptibility to contamination by the protein component of tears. As mentioned above, for high oxygen transmissibility through a hydrogel contact lens, an alternative to high water content is to make a thinner lens of a relatively lower hydration. These lenses may have improved mechanical and optical performance, as well as more resistance to contamination. The development of CSI (crofilcon A) contact lenses of Corneal Sciences Inc. was based on this principle. These lenses are made of a copolymer of glycerol monomethacrylate with methyl methacrylate.

Hydrogel lenses of lower hydration than the original poly(hydroxyethyl methacrylate) hydrogel lenses are made by copolymerizing hydroxyethyl methacrylate with a relatively hydrophobic monomer. Thus, Gelflex (dimefilcon A) of Calcon Laboratories is a copolymer of hydroxyethyl methacrylate with methyl methacrylate and ethylene bis-(oxyethylene) dimethacrylate as the cross-linking agent. A copolymer of hydroxyethyl methacrylate with ethoxyethyl methacrylate is used in the DuraSoft (phemfilcon A) contact lenses of Wesley-Jessen, Inc.

Corneal Prosthesis

Transplantation of a cornea from a donor eye to a recipient eye (keratoplasty) is very often successful. However, eyes with certain unfavorable corneal lesions usually respond poorly to keratoplasty. In such cases, an artificial plastic cornea or keratoprosthesis offers the only hope to obtain some temporary or permanent improvement of vision. A corneal plastic implant consists essentially of a cylindrical portion that penetrates "through-and-through" the cornea. The optical cylinder is usually held in place by means of an intralamellar flange with perforations for the ingrowth of tissue, but there are many different models of keratoprosthesis, one of the most common being the so-called collar-button type corneal prosthesis [9].

The material most commonly used for artificial corneal implants is poly(methyl methacrylate), particularly for the optical cylinder or optical

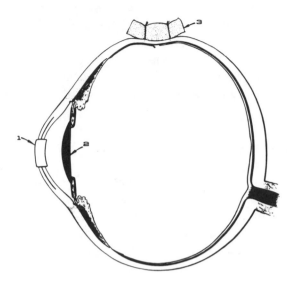

Figure 2. Schematic representation of an eye with (1) a keratoprosthesis, (2) an artificial intraocular lens, and (3) an episcleral implant for scleral buckling of retinal detachment.

portion of the prosthesis. The supporting flange has been made of a variety of materials ranging from Dacron or Teflon fabric to tooth or bone.

Itoi et al. [10] experimented with corneal prostheses made of a hydrogel consisting of complexes of poly(vinyl alcohol) with poly(acrylic acid), but these were found to opacify after implantation.

It is this author's experience that hydrogels in general are poor materials for incompletely covered corneal prostheses, because dehydration and shrinkage will dislodge the prosthesis from the tissues. Therefore, through-and-through keratoprostheses were lathe-cut from hydrophilic acrylic xerogels. These were implanted in rabbit corneas under conjunctival flaps and allowed to swell. These prostheses, made of poly(hydroxyethyl methacrylate) or poly(glyceryl methacrylate-co-methyl methacrylate), swelled isotropically about 18% linear dimension, and it was hoped that, upon swelling, they would lock tightly against the surrounding tissue, thereby avoiding the problem of extrusion so common with corneal prostheses. However, these hydrogel prostheses extruded from the cornea during swelling. Another problem related to the possible use of any type of hydrogel for an incompletely covered type of implant, such as a keratoprosthesis, is that hydrogels are prone to contamination with protein and other deposits. These problems are relatively easy to avoid in hydrogel contact lenses by periodic cleaning, i.e., protein deposits on hydrogel contact lenses are usually removed by treating the lenses with the enzyme papain. However, with a corneal implant *in situ,* this would not be possible.

Intraocular Lens Implants

Opacification of the crystalline lens of the eye due to disease or trauma is a cataract. When a cataract is removed surgically, light can reach the retina again, but, for the aphakic patient to see once more, an optical correction must be provided. The optical correction can be in the form of spectacle lenses, a contact lens, or an intraocular artificial plastic lens. Intraocular artificial lens implant surgery recently has become a relatively common operation.

In 1960 Dreifus et al. [11] proposed the use of nonionizable neutral hydrocolloid acrylates (glycol methacrylate hydrogels) as intraocular lenses, and enumerated the possible advantages of these materials over poly(methyl methacrylate) and other materials used as intraocular lenses. However, poly(methyl methacrylate) is today the only material used for the intraocular lens implants. Some models of lenses have had some supporting loops or flanges made of polypropylene or some other material, but poly(methyl methacrylate) has always been used for the optical and major part of the implant.

Poly(methyl methacrylate) is very well tolerated by eye tissues. However, its purity is not easy to ascertain. One property of this polymer is that it depolymerizes during mechanical working, such as machining and polishing, so that even when the original material is of the highest degree of purity (such as medical grade Perspex), it is not always possible to know the purity of the finished implant. Nevertheless, most complications of intraocular lenses usually result from surgical trauma, such as accidental contact of the implant with the delicate endothelial cellular layer on the back of the cornea, rather than to reaction to the plastic itself.

In general, short-term results (up to several years) with intraocular lenses have been good. However, ophthalmologists are proceeding with caution because they are uncertain about the long-term effects that an artificial lens might have on the corneal endothelium and retina [12].

Glaucoma Drainage Devices

Glaucoma is a condition marked by increased intraocular pressure, which, if not treated, leads to blindness. In certain glaucoma conditions that do not respond to more conservative medical or surgical treatment, tubes are implanted to drain aqueous humor. Usually, one end of the tube is placed in the anterior chamber of the eye and the other end drains into the subconjunctiva or suprachoroidal spaces. Unfortunately, the relief of intraocular pressure is often only temporary, because the tubes tend to become occluded by fibrous proliferation around the part of the implant embedded in tissue.

One of the most successful drainage devices for glaucoma is a strip made of poly(hydroxyethyl methacrylate) hydrogel that contains parallel capillary-size channels through it. The dry implant is partially inserted in the anterior chamber. The strip swells on hydration to plug the surgical incision. The capillary channels in the strip and the filtering bleb permit slow drainage of fluid to the subconjunctiva [13].

Scleral Buckling in Retinal Detachment Surgery

The retina is the innermost cellular layer on the posterior portion of the eye, and it is the part of the eye where light perception takes place. When the retina detaches from the underlying choroidal layer, light perception on the detached portion of retina ceases. The object of retinal detachment surgery is to restore light perception by reattaching the detached retina and its nutrition source at the choroidal layer. This can be accomplished by pushing the retina back from the vitreous cavity by means of an injectable substance or with a device such as an intraocular balloon, and/or most commonly, by buckling the wall of the eye over the area of the detached retina by means of a scleral implant. The scleral implant will also relieve the tension on the retina caused by a shrinking vitreous body [14].

Many materials have been employed for scleral buckling in retinal detachment surgery. Currently, the most commonly used materials are silicone rubber and sponge for nonabsorbable implants in permanent scleral buckles and absorbable gelatin for temporary scleral buckles. The potential of acrylic hydrogels for use as scleral buckling material in retinal detachment surgery was recognized early by Wichterle and coworkers [15]. They used poly(hydroxyethyl methacrylate) hydrogel rods rein-

forced with polyester fiber in short-term animal experiments that compared the hydrogel with the commonly used silicone rubber.

High scleral indentation can be obtained with hydrophilic insoluble
polymers, which are implanted in the dry state (xerogels) and then ex-
pand by imbibing tissue fluid. Absorbable gelatin, nonabsorbable
poly(hydroxyethyl methacrylate), and poly(glyceryl methacrylate) have
been implanted as xerogels in scleral buckling procedures. Two different
gels were made from glyceryl methacrylate by varying the concentration
of the monomer in the prepolymer mixture. A dilute mixture (12 parts
water to 1 part monomer) produced a polymer that was a very soft gel
when hydrated. A more concentrated mixture (5 parts water to 1 part
monomer) formed a hydrogel that had the consistency of soft rubber.
Homogeneous hydroxyethyl methacrylate hydrogels exhibited a relatively constant degree of swelling regardless of the initial prepolymerization
dilution. This hydrogel is rubbery but firmer than poly(glyceryl
methacrylate) 5:1. Animal experiments with these hydrogels showed
them to be promising nonabsorbable materials for scleral buckling [16].
Hydrated poly(glyceryl methacrylate) 5:1 is softer than silicone rubber,
and will adapt to variations in intraocular pressure. Hydrated
poly(hydroxyethyl methacrylate) is firmer than the silicone rubber used in
retina surgery and will not readily yield to changes in intraocular
pressure. Poly(glyceryl methacrylate) 12:1 is too soft, when hydrated, to
produce a buckling effect. The animal experiments were followed by
operation on 24 humans with retinal detachment. Xerogels of
poly(glyceryl methacrylate) 5:1 were implanted intrasclerally, resulting in
a marked sclerochoroidal indentation by swelling of the implant [17].

Gelatin, poly(hydroxyethyl methacrylate), and poly(glyceryl
methacrylate) are soft when hydrated, but are hard and brittle in the
dehydrated state. However, poly(hydroxyethyl acrylate) is soft not only
when hydrated but also when dehydrated. Dry poly(hydroxyethyl
acrylate) can be carved easily to shape and size, and, because it is soft, it
might be very useful for operations on thin, weakened sclera. Animal experiments have shown that poly(hydroxyethyl acrylate) hydrogels are as
nontoxic and well tolerated as other materials in clinical use. Another advantage of hydrogels over other implant materials is that they can easily
be impregnated with aqueous antibiotics to achieve prolonged antibiotic
delivery to the surgical site [18].

Vitreous Implants

A vitreous supplement is a useful adjunct in some types of retina surgery, particularly in the management of complex cases. The many substances that have been used for this purpose are of two types: (1) absorbable fluids and gases, and (2) nonabsorbable fluids, gels, and balloons. Silicone oil has been widely used as a permanent vitreous supplement, but it has been found unsatisfactory on long-term observation. Hyaluronic acid, a component of the extracellular matrix of connective tissue such as the vitreous, subcutaneous tissue, umbilical cord, synovial fluid, etc, is currently used with good results as a temporary vitreous supplement in special cases [19].

Poly(glyceryl methacrylate) 12:1 hydrogel has proved to be well tolerated in eyes of experimental animals. The consistency of the hydrogels depends on their degree of hydration, and the density of the most highly hydrated gels is slightly above that of water. These hydrogels are very soft and optically clear with a refractive index very close to that of the natural vitreous. An important property of a highly hydrated gel (about 98-99% water), in reference to its application as a vitreous implant, is the large decrease in volume that occurs when the gel is completely dehydrated. The dehydrated gel is implanted in the vitreous cavity and expands upon absorbing liquid vitreous, or physiological saline that is injected at the time of gel implantation. The main problems encountered concerned implantation technique, because, although the dehydrated gel was relatively small, it was at least 3 mm in diameter and difficult to place into the vitreous cavity. An alternative method to implantation of a formed hydrogel into the vitreous cavity is to implant a gel that has been cast in a cylindrical shape, and then to inject it to full hydration with a suitable injecting device, preferably tubular in shape with a gradually narrowing funnel-like end (rather than with the usual syringe and needle which will fragment the gel). Based on visual acuity and light transmission tests, implantable cylindrical gels of the largest diameter possible provide the best transparency. The fragmented gels obtained by injecting the hydrogel through a needle provide the poorest optical medium and are the least transparent material [20].

Wichterle and coworkers used lightly cross-linked hydrogels obtained from methacrylic acid and glycerol. If a strong mineral acid is used for the esterification, this reaction is immediately followed by the polymerization reaction, because a strongly acidic medium greatly accelerates the polymerization, particularly that of monomers of the acrylic and methacrylic series. According to Wichterle, at a water content above 95%, the gels are sufficiently optically homogeneous and can be squeezed even by means of thin injection needles, which greatly simplifies the operation technique. These gels were applied in experimental animals and in humans, in the partial or total exchange of the vitreous body [21].

REFERENCES

1. Ray, G.S., van Heuven, W.A.J., and Patel, D: Gelatin implants in scleral buckling procedures. Arch Ophthalmol 93:799-802, 1975.
2. Schepens, C.L., Okamura, I.D., Brockhurst, R.J., and Regan, C.D.J.: Scleral buckling procedures. V. Synthetic sutures and silicone implants. Arch Ophthalmol 64:868-881, 1960.
3. Thomas, W.M.: Acrylamide polymers. *In* Encyclopedia of Polymer Science and Technology: Plastics, Resins, Rubbers, Fibers. New York, Interscience, vol. 1, pp. 177-197, 1964.
4. Wichterle, O., and Lim, D.: Hydrophilic gels for biological use. Nature 185:117-118, 1960.
5. Andrade, J.D. (ed): Hydrogels for medical and related applications. ACS Symposium Series 31, American Chemical Society, Washington, D.C., 1976.
6. Refojo, M.F.: Materials for use in the eye. *In* Polymers in Medicine and Surgery. Kronenthal, R.L., Oser, Z., and Martin E. (eds), Polymer Science and Technology, vol. 8., New York, Plenum Press, pp. 313-331, 1975.
7. Refojo, M.F.: Contact lenses. *In* Encyclopedia of Polymer Science and Technology. Bikales, N.M. (ed), New York, John Wiley, Suppl. 1, pp. 195-219, 1976.
8. Refojo, M.F.: Contact lenses. *In* Kirk/Othmer Encyclopedia of Chemical Technology, 3rd ed. New York, Wiley-Interscience, 1979, vol. 6, pp. 720-742.
9. Symposium: Keratoprosthesis. Trans Am Acad Ophthalmol Otolaryngol 83 (2): OP249-OP282, 1977.
10. Itoi, M., Akiyama, T., Komatsu, S., and Niwa, Y.: Experimental study of elastic keratoprosthesis: A preliminary report. Jpn J Ophthalmol 9:146-149, 1965.
11. Dreifus, M., Wichterle, O., and Lim, D.: [Intra-cameral lenses made of hydrocolloidal acrylates.] Cesk Oftalmol 16:154-159, 1960. (Cz).
12. Symposium: Intraocular lenses. Trans Am Acad Ophthalmol Otolaryngol 81(1):OP64-OP137, 1976.
13. Krejci, L., Harrison, R., and Wichterle, O.: Hydroxyethyl methacrylate capillary strip. Animal trials with a new glaucoma drainage device. Arch Ophthalmol 84:76-82, 1970.
14. Pruett, R.C., and Regan, C.D.J. (eds,): Retina Congress. New York, Appleton-Century-Crofts, 1974.
15. Kristek, A., König, B., and Wichterle, O.: [Contribution to the surgery of retinal detachment.] Cesk Oftalmol 22:58-61, 1966. (Cz).

16. Calabria, G.A., Pruett, R.C., and Refojo, M.F.: Further experience with sutureless scleral buckling materials. I. Hydrogels. Arch Ophthalmol 86:77-81, 1971.
17. Grignolo, A., Refojo, M.F., Calabria, G.A., and Zingirian, M.: L'emploi des hydrogels synthetiques dans la chirurgie du decollement de la retine. Mod Probl Ophthalmol 10:153-159, 1972.
18. Refojo, M.F., and Liu, H.S.: Experimental scleral buckling with a soft xerogel implant. I. Properties of poly(hydroxyethyl acrylate) compared with gelatin and other swelling implants. Ophthalmic Surg 9(6):43-50, 1978. II. Experiments in vivo. *ibid.* 10(11):52-56, 1979.
19. Tolentino, F.I., Schepens, C.L., and Freeman, H.M.: Vitreoretinal Disorders, Diagnosis and Management. Philadelphia, W.B. Saunders, pp. 490-511, 1976.
20. Refojo, M.F., and Zauberman, H.: Optical properties of gels designed for vitreous implantation. Invest Ophthalmol 12:465-467, 1973.
21. Medical Polymers: Chemical Problems. Institute of Macromolecular Chemistry, 17th Microsymposium on Macromolecules. Prague, Aug. 15-18, 1977. J Polym Sci Polymer Symp 66, 1979.

CONSIDERATIONS ON ENCAPSULATION FOR ACUTE/CHRONIC LONGEVITY OF ELECTRONIC IMPLANTS

John W. Boretos

Biomedical Engineering and Instrumentation Branch
Division of Research Services
National Institutes of Health
Bethesda, Maryland 20014

INTRODUCTION

Encapsulated electronic implants must function under the same acute/long-term constraints associated with other prosthetic devices. Because of their nature, however, they have unique breakdown problems which have been the focus of interest in recent years as demand for these devices has grown. The artificial pacemaker, for example, is one of the most outstanding accomplishments in the field of surgical implants with literally thousands of units in service. Although they have a 20-year history of satisfactory performance, premature failures still occur. To counter these difficulties is not easily accomplished. The basic chemical physical criteria for encapsulation have long been established by the electronics industry, but the application of such systems to *in vivo* use puts more stringent demands on the materials and allows less latitude in the manner in which they can be handled. Meeting the requirements for acceptable performance has been largely empirical in nature due to a host of complicating factors which serve to mediate the ultimate behavior and usually can not be predicted, *a priori*, for each new situation. A system optimized for one particular application may be useless or harmful in another, depending upon the area of the body in which the device is to be used. Consideration must be given to physically stabilizing the device and minimizing bulk to preclude ulceration through the skin. Often, maintenance of nutrient supply to surrounding tissue and cellular response at the tissue/implant interface are determining factors in achieving acceptability and longevity. Many materials are inherently unsuitable as encapsulants when subject to the living environment. They may be excessively permeable to body moisture and salts which can lead to critical shifts in electrical signals; they may degrade into lower molecular weight components which can change the physical properties or chemical stability as first observed; or they may exude impurities which can produce adverse cellular responses. Because of these and numerous other uncertainties, tripartite interactions between encapsulating materials, tissues, and devices have been the subject of considerable investigation. This paper discusses those aspects of encapsulation that have consistently caused the greatest degree of difficulty with electronic implants and surveys the materials and methods that produce the best results.

MATERIALS AND METHODS FOR INCREASED PERFORMANCE

Physiological Considerations

No artificial material is completely inert or ideal as an encapsulating material. In general, man-made substances are subject to unfavorable alteration or interaction in the body depending upon the physical, chemical and electrical stresses to which they are exposed and the duration of implantation. The extent to which this alteration occurs largely determines the suitability for specific applications.

In selecting an encapsulant for acute or chronic use, physiological interaction with tissues becomes a major consideration. Some materials function satisfactorily for a few days or weeks before chemical or physical changes induce irritation. If the device is intended to be placed in the blood stream, it can generate thrombi and small clots which may be transported throughout the vascular system. To retard thrombus formation, it is generally agreed that surfaces must be smooth and clean, and the configuration must avoid contours which encourage stasis, stagnation, or turbulence of the blood. Attempts to modify surfaces to minimize thrombogenicity have met with varying degrees of success, but few have been applied to electronic devices.

Mechanical Considerations

Adverse reactions can be generated by mechanical shortcomings. Shape, size, and weight depend crucially upon the particular site selected for the implant. Nerves, blood vessels, and other tissues are easily damaged by undue force or pressure exerted by sharp corners, protrusions or abrasive surfaces. Erosion through the skin and excessive keratin formation have been observed as a result of improperly secured implants or the presence of dead space around the implant which can permit migration of the device. Because of their geometry, cylinders exhibit a tendency to shift orientation and migrate; disks, on the other hand, are less mobile. Sharp angles are responsible for fibrous capsular thickening and the presence of excessive interstitial tissue substance which are almost absent at smooth, round rims. Epithelial encapsulation has been generally observed only in implants which do not have acute angles.

Permeability Considerations

The need to protect implantable electronic devices from the wet environment of the body has fostered a number of studies [1-15] into the suitability of various encapsulants and combinations thereof. These have encompassed both coating and casting compounds of such diverse substances as silicone rubber, silicone rubber/wax combinations, polyolefin/wax combinations, waxes, varnishes, poly (methyl methacrylate), natural rubber impregnated with silicone grease, polyvinyl chloride paints, vapor deposited paraxylylene, ceramics and cast epoxies. Most of these substances have used an overcoat of silicone rubber to impart additional moisture resistance and improved tissue compatibility.

Organic materials, often thought to be "waterproof", do transmit water to varying degrees. Table 1 ranks the commonly considered materials in order of their individual permeabilities; they will all eventually reach a state of equilibrium with the surrounding environment. There is no direct relationship between the amount that permeates, that which is absorbed, and the deterioration of the polymer during immersion. Some materials, such as poly (methyl methacrylate), silicone rubber, and the various epoxies, have relatively high permeability to moisture but are important because they can be readily cast or used as a coating, whereas materials with extremely low moisture vapor transmission rates are usually only available as pre-cast films.

Table 1. *Moisture Vapor Transmission of Several Polymers [16].*

Polymer (2 mil film)	Moisture Vapor Transmission (measured at 30.8 C and 90-98% RH) g-mil/100 in^2-24 hr
Polymonochlorotrifluroethylene	0.02
Ethylene/vinyl acetate	0.20
Polyvinylidene chloride	1
Para-xylylene	1
Epoxy	2
Polypropylene	0.7-3.0
Polytetrafluoroethylene	3
Polyurethanes*	2-9
Polycarbonate	10
Polyethylene	21
Polymethyl methacrylate	35
Polyethylene terephthalate	48
Polystyrene	120
Cellophane	134
Silicone rubber	170

*Depends on type

Corrosion Considerations

Water is implicated in the failure of electronic implants because it provides the environment necessary for corrosive breakdown of the circuitry. The degree to which corrosion occurs depends upon the presence of chloride and other ions, the type of metallic components used, the amount of moisture present and the interfacial bond strength of the encapsulating system. If an ionizable impurity is present on or near the surface, conductive media is produced as moisture solvates it. Thereupon, conductive pathways may short circuit the unit or electrical resistance may actually be increased due to the formation of corrosion deposits. Typical examples of such contaminants would be solder fluxes (especially activated fluxes containing a halogen), body salts (usually from fingerprints) and residues from chlorinated cleaning solutions absorbed into and held by the plastic components. The choice of metals used for the circuitry often influences reliability. For example, silver and copper are especially susceptible to electrolyte corrosion and can produce metallic dendrites. Metal growths known as dendrites can occur between two metallic conductors that are separated by an insulator and subject to an applied voltage. When the resistance of the insulator is degraded, in the presence of water, a form of electrodeposition can take place if the corrosion products of the anode are sufficiently ionized and mobile to migrate to the cathode under the influence of the electrical field. As more and more ions are deposited, a preference for the site of initial deposition encourages further growth of the dendrite until a bridge is formed between the positive and negative charged areas [17].

Use of Conformal Coatings

Conformal coatings are attractive to the electronics designer. Aside from the fact that they do not add appreciably to the weight or bulk of the unit, the major value lies in their ability to act as a moisture and gas barrier to prevent corrosion and electrical breakdown. Significant in achieving this goal is (a) the "wet-resistance" of the substance, (b) the level of adhesion of the coating/substrate interface and (c) the ability of the substrates to form layers free of pin-holes. Most materials fail as conformal coatings because of their inability to completely cover corners and edges. Vapor deposited Parylene C [18] excels in achieving non-porous and uniformly coated surfaces — even over "knife-edges." The polymer is the product of the dimer, dichloro-di-para-xylene, which is vaporized at elevated temperatures to form the monomer, chloro-para xylene. The molecular cloud thus formed can be introduced into a deposition chamber where it condenses evenly on all exposed surfaces (at room temperature). Polymerization occurs spontaneously on substrate surfaces and precludes potential impurities and in-homogenieties in film structure foam forming. The coating has the further advantage of exerting no distorting forces on the substrate at any thickness (2-3 mils maximum).

Loeb and coworkers [19] reported that a 3 micron thick coating of Parylene-C over "1-2 megohm iridium microelectrodes" has prevented significant impedance changes for over four months in a monkey's brain. However, Thornton [20] describes tests where he coated resistors with various substances and measured the time in saline before the resistances had dropped to 75 percent of the original value. In his test, Silastic 382RTV [21], Silastic with 15 percent beeswax, and a mixture of wax/Elvax (85/15) performed considerably better than the Parylene-C. Perhaps this was due in part to the relative "wet-resistance" of the compounds tested.

Certainly, a significant drawback to the use of para-xylene for moisture protection is its lack of adhesion to the substrates which it coats. There is no chemical interaction with most surfaces, since the paraxylene molecules react chemically only with each other.

Other materials such as ceramics have been used as conformal coatings for electronic circuitry with considerable success. Wise and Weissman [22] describe the use of thin films of glass for protecting integrated circuits for use in biological systems and reports the technique particularly suitable for insulating microelectrodes. Films of silicon dioxide and silicon nitride, 0.2-0.3 millimicrons thick, exhibit excellent corrosion protection for unencapsulated transistors implanted in the brain for periods of up to 4 months. These glassy films can be achieved using various means, i.e., pyrolytic deposition, vacuum evaporation and sputtering; however, thermally sensitive substances to be coated could be adversely affected by the high temperature essential to the processes.

Use of Potting Compounds

Although "potting" techniques are simple in principle, difficulties are encountered in obtaining void-free castings with negligible shrinkage, low heats of reaction, and complete polymerization. To achieve high density castings, the units should be degassed under vacuum prior to and immediately after the potting material is poured to eliminate entrained air. If rigid encapsulating materials are used and the shrinkage values are high, breakage of fine wires or shifting of operating characteristics can result. The great variety of available casting resins and curing agents allow for a wide range of compositions and properties to match most specifications. The epoxies, especially those crosslinked with an aromatic amine or an anhydride, offer the best moisture resistance. The earliest cardiac pacemakers designed by Kantrowitz [4] and Zoll [2] used such systems and continue in commercial use today. Critchfield and associates [23] found that packages encapsulated with epoxy-Silastic® and epoxy-glass-Silastic® layers require as much as ten times the volume of the circuitry to afford reasonable protection from body fluid penetrations. However, recent advances in quality control have allowed considerable reduction in bulk. For medical use, bisphenol A type epoxies catalyzed with diethylenetriamine (DETA) have a dependable record of service. Two such compounds are listed in Table 2 along with their typical properties. If these substances are carefully checked from batch to batch to assure that their quality is comparable with values taken from original qualifying batches and thereafter carefully combined in stoichometric amounts with minimum inclusion of microvoids during casting followed by a complete curing cycle, experience has shown that tissue acceptability will be high and moisture uptake will be limited to 2-4 weight percent over a 30 month period [24].

Table 2. Typical Epoxy Systems Used for Encapsulating Electronic Implants.

Resin	Cure	Water Absorption, 24 hrs. immersion, percent*	Dielectric Strength, volts/mil	Typical Linear Shrinkage in/in
Scotchcast #5** with DETA	1 hr @ 60°C to 24 hrs @ 23°C	--	325	0.004
Hysol R8-2083*** with curing agent #H-2-3475	2 hrs @ 60°	0.15	563	0.004

*   The Scotchcast shows about 2% by weight moisture uptake at 37°C over 30 months, Hysol shows about a 4% gain (24).
**   Minnesota Mining and Manufacturing Co., St. Paul, Minnesota.
*** Hysol Corp., Olean, NY.

Salyer and coworkers [25] devised a composite system of epoxy and urethane which shows good thromboresistance. Pluronic F-68, a non-ionic degergent, and heparin have alternatively been included in rigid, semi-flexible and flexible formulations to achieve improved blood compatibility. Although these compounds have been shown to be useful for components of circulatory assist devices, no experience with their use as encapsulants has been reported.

Conductive epoxy resin mixtures with low resistivity fillers such as silver, gold, etc., are being used in place of solder in some areas to overcome corrosion difficulties. Typically, they exhibit volume resistivities in the order of 2×10^{-4} ohm-cm [26]. Ceramic capacitors are usually provided with metal filled conductive epoxy ends to provide mechanical and electrical connection. Redemski [27] suggests that attachment of integrated circuits by means of conductive epoxy provides a beneficial amount of thermal conductivity even when not required for electrical connection. Transistors and diodes that do pass current can use the conductive epoxy if a gold backing is present to prevent ohmic drift.

As previously mentioned, silicone rubber has been widely used as a conformal coating and as a potting compound to protect electronic components. The most popular form of this versatile material for insulating electronics is the room temperature vulcanizing (RTV) variety.

Room temperature vulcanizing compounds are liquids and pastes that cure to solid, resilient elastomers. They can be subdivided into two groups: (a) the single component system and (b) the two component system. The former is familiar in the squeeze tube form (Silastic® Medical Adhesive Type A). In the single component system hydroxyl terminated methyl siloxane is present with methyl triacetoxysilane. When the mixture is exposed to moisture from the air, the acetoxy groups are cleared from the methyl triacetoxysilane and transformed into volatile acetic acid and methylsilane having multiple hydroxyl groups. The latter spontaneously combines with the hydroxyl terminated methylsilane present to extend the polymer chain and to form suitable crosslinks. Raw silicone rubber readily bonds to other silicones and provides a convenient adhesive. In the two component system, e.g. the potting compound Silastic® 382, hydroxyl terminated methyl-siloxane is packaged in combination withpropylorthosilicate as one component. With the addition of the second component, the catalyst, the hydroxyl groups react to split off the alkyl groups, and the polymer is then available to crosslink through the remaining silicate.

The common use of numerous additives to achieve specific properties in most industrial elastomers is precluded by the potentially adverse effects of eluting components. In tailoring silicones for medical use, the approach has been to minimize complications by keeping the system as simple as inert as possible. Crosslinking agents must be chosen carefully since they influence the properties of the finished rubber. Reinforcing agents are necessary in silicone rubber formulations to provide strength and bulk. For example, the tensile strength of a vulcanized gum can be increased from 100 psi to over 1200 psi with proper compounding. Diatomaceous earths are incorporated into the RTV potting compounds because they possess an excellent balance of handling properties and strength for these liquid systems. To add radiopaque qualities to silicone rubber, barium sulfate can be "milled" into the various types.

Use of Hermetic Seals

Moisture can be found in many places within a pacemaker before and after implantation. The amount depends upon the conditions to which the individual components and the unit as a whole have been subjected. Ferreira [28] describes five mechanisms by which moisture reaches the units: (1) moisture entering through the epoxy or silicone rubber encapsulating material, (2) moisture trapped in the free space of the units, (3) moisture sealed in the batteries, (4) moisture trapped in the electronic components or in the circuit enclosures and (5) moisture entering the electronic enclosure. For these reasons, Thompson (29) attempted to develop hermetically sealed units that would remain completely free from the influence of moisture by enveloping them in a stainless steel can filled to within 1/16 inch of the top with silicone rubber and closed with a heliac welded lid.

The development and commercial use of non-gassing lithium cells, the use of "getters," the development of rechargeability, single cell circuitry and sophisticated welding techniques make the concept of a totally enclosed, hermetically-sealed unit feasible. However, a number of perplexing problems are associated with the otherwise simple concept of isolating diverse circuitry in a metallic can.

Current hermetically sealed pulse generators consist of a lithium battery, electronic circuitry and the pulse generator package. The interconnecting areas contain discrete components, feedthroughs and soldered or welded connections which are subject to moisture related failure mechanisms. Therefore, the various components must be baked at 250°C for 10 hours to remove most of the moisture and the assembly carried on in a dry atmosphere without exposure to the atmosphere for even a few seconds [30]. This produces a package having a relatively safe total water content (1000 ppm). However, lower temperatures (i.e. 125°C) and exposure to short intervals at ambient conditions raise moisture levels from 800 to 5400 ppm as measured by mass-spectrometry. Epoxy backfill has been used to serve as a secondary barrier within the hermetically sealed case in the event that the case should leak. The disadvantages somewhat outweigh the advantages in this latter approach. Namely, the epoxy filler adds additional weight, entails adverse shrinkage and makes analysis difficult after failure. Redimski [26] suggests that after a drying regimen similar to that above, the cured unit should be further baked at 155-160°C for one hour to insure complete cross-linking. He further recommends that epoxy material for use in hybrid components should follow these guidelines: (1) primary or secondary amine curing agents should be avoided; single system epoxies are desirable; (2) no outgassing should occur below 200°C and (3) no chemical reactions should occur below 200°C.

Sealing of the metal cases is usually accomplished by any of four welding techniques: (1) plasma arc, (2) gas tungsten arc, (3) laser process, or (4) electron beam process [31]. Even though the heat of the weld is largely limited to the weld joint in these techniques, any polymeric material accidentally entrapped in the weld joint can generate a pin-hole and destroy the integrity.

Simple circuits have been shown to function satisfactorily up to 18 months when hermetically sealed in soft glass [32]. However, the temperature needed to melt the glass causes a random permanent shift of the frequency and therefore results in a reduced yield. The use of batteries or active circuitry together with this type of hermetic sealing appears to be impractical at present.

The Importance of Cleaning

Cleanliness is essential throughout all stages of an electronic implant's preparation and is effort well invested in preventing subsequent malfunctions. The best measures preclude the use of oily materials, soldering acids, salt contaminants, and other foreign substances. However, in many instances suitable cleaning procedures are required. Commercial cleaning fluids for use on switches, potentiometer tracks, and electrical contacts may contain toxic chlorinated hydrocarbons and therefore should be used with care or not at all. A spray arrangement used in a well ventilated hood is an efficient means of mechanically scrubbing and removing debris from otherwise inaccessible areas. Teflon® and nylon insulation are particularly difficult to clean because of their porous structure.

Gilman reports [33] that the adhesion of an epoxy encapsulant, and thus its ability to inhibit corrosive forces as previously discussed, is directly related to the cleanliness of the surfaces which it contacts. The cleaner the surface, the more readily the epoxy will "wet" the surface the bond will be.

Testing as a Tool

Testing of electronic implants is an important aspect of their manufacture. Not only does testing provide an important means of quality control, but it also produces valuable information about long-term performance and furnishes a means by which various investigators may compare results. Several such tests have been established as standards by the American Society for Testing and Materials Committee F-1 on Electronics [34].

ASTM Commiteee F-1 on Electronics Standards

F-74 Hydrolytic Stability of Plastic Encapsulants

F-100 Shrinkage Stresses in Plastic Embedment Materials

F-135 Embedment Stress Caused by Casting Compounds

8C06 Completeness of Cure of Encapsulants

8C26 Microcircuit Coatings, Evaluating

8C33 Transfer Moulding Compounds for Encapsulation

Tests [35] to determine hermeticity of an implant package are summarized as follows:

Bubble Test: A visual inspection of bubbles escaping from the package when immersed in a hot fluorocarbon.

Pressure Bubble Test: A visual inspection of bubbles escaping after an immersion in low-boiling fluid under pressure followed by a heated fluid.

Weight Gain: Measured weight increase after immersion in a liquid under pressure.

Differential Pressure Method (for large volume packages): The package is evacuated in one chamber (whereupon an interconnecting source chamber at known integral gas pressure is connected to the test chamber by opening a valve. A gross leak is indicated if the pressure in the combined volume is lower than expected for the volumes of the package, the source, and test chamber. A growing differential pressure between the two chambers indicates a small leak and may be calculated.

Helium Leak Detector Method (Indirect mode): The package is pressurized under helium after which any escaping helium coming out of the package can be detected with a mass spectrometer.

Helium Leak Detector Method (Direct Mode):

   Prefill Procedure: The package is sealed in a helium atmosphere, and any leak escaping from the unit is measured.

   Flush Procedure: A vent which is part of the package is connected to a mass spectrometer to detect the penetration of any helium that is used to flush the outside of the package.

Radioisotope Method: The package is pressurized in an atmosphere of Krypton-85, and the leak rate is measured with a scintillation counter to detect any radioactive gas inside.

Although these tests are of significant value, Thomas [30] describes a situation where devices have passed a helium fine leak and gross bubble test as specified by MIL-STD-883A only to fail after 50 hours of operation due to short circuits brought on by moisture induced gold migration. The thermal shock test specified in the qualification procedure and its subsequent quenching had fractured a glass-to-metal seal and allowed water vapor to enter the interior of the package.

To further complicate the testing data, Ruthberg [36] points out that a definitive gas leak rate pertinent to moisture ingress is not available, and it is difficult to predict the rate by which moisture will enter a container characterized by a given leak (See Schafft [35] for leak rate defined).

CONCLUSIONS

After 20 years of experience with various telemetry devices, the number of suitable materials consists essentially of those same materials initially considered, namely, the epoxies and silicone rubber. However, much has been done to optimize their properties and performance by controlling purity, quality and processing conditons. Although exotic materials such as paraxylylene and inorganic oxides seem suitable for some applications, they are limited for many others. Polymeric encapsulants lack the necessary properties to serve as permanent barriers to the physiological environment and as such have not been optimum for long-term uninterrupted control over vital body functions. Consequently, industry has placed recent emphasis on total hermeticity via welded cases over the electronic circuitry.

REFERENCES

1.   Chardack, W.M., Gage, A.A., and Greatbach, W.A.: *Surgery* 48:643, 1960.
2.   Zoll, P.M., Frank, H.A., Zarsky, L.R.N., Linenthal, A.J., and Belgard, A.H.: *Annals of Surg.* 154: 330, 1961.
3.   Hawthorne, E.W. and Harvey, E.J.: *Appl. Physiol.* 16:6, 1961.
4.   Kantrowitz, A., Cohen, R., Heinz, R., Schmidt, T. and Feldman, D.S.: *Surgery, Gynecology and Obstetrics,* 115:415, 1962.

5. Levitsky, S., Glenn, W.W.L., Mauro, A., Eisenberg, L., and Smoth, P.W.: *Surgery* 52:64, 1961.
6. McCoy, E.L. and Bass, P.: *Amer. J. Physiol.* 205:439, 1963.
7. Bradley, W.E., Chou, S.N., and French, L.A.: *J. of Neurosurg.* 20:953, 1963.
8. Bassett, A.L., Pawluk, R.J., and Becker, R.O.: *Nature* 204:652, 1964.
9. Kantrowitz, A. and Schamaum, M.: *JAMA* 187:127, 1964.
10. Balin, H., Busser, J.H., Hatke, F., Fromm, E., Wan, L.S., and Israel, S.L.: *Obstet. Gynec.* 24:198, 1964.
11. deVilliers, R., Nose, Y., Meier, W., and Kantrowitz, A.: *Trans. Amer. Soc. Artif. Intern. Organs* 10:357, 1964.
12. Mackay, R. Stuart: *Biomedical Telemetry, Sensing and Transmitting Biological Information from Animal and Man.* New York, Wiley Publishing Co., 1968.
13. Reininger, E.J. and Hinchey, E.J.: *J. Appl. Physio.* 24:580, 1968.
14. Frank, H.A., Zoll, P.M., and Linenthal, A.J.: *J. of Thorac. Cardiovasc. Surg.* 57:17, 1969.
15. Goodman, R.M. and Gibson, R.J.: *Bioscience* 20:19, 1970.
16. Boretos, J.W.: IEEE Transactions on Industrial Electronics and Control Instrumentation, *IECI-17:* 151, 1970.
17. Frankenthal, R.P.: Semiconductor Measurement Technology: Reliability Technology for Cardiac Pacemakers III-A Workshop Report. USDC/NBS Special Pub. #400-42, p. 12, Aug. 1977.
18. "Union Carbide Process Data, Bakelite Parylene General Information." Union Carbide Corp., New York.
19. Loeb, G.E. Bak, M.J., Salcman, M. and Schmidt, E.M.: *IEEE Trans. on Biomedical Engr.* 2:121, 1977.
20. Thornton, A.: Reliability Technology for Cardiac Pacemakers III. USDC/NBS Proceedings Workshop III, p. 47, Oct. 1977.
21. Dow Corning Corp., Midland, Michigan.
22. Wise, K.D. and Weissman, R.H.: *Med. & Biol. Engr.* 9:339, 1971.
23. Critchfield, F.H. Jr., Critchfield, F.H., Neuman, M.R. and Lin, K.Y.: *Proc. 21st Ann. Conf. on Engr. in Med. & Biol.* 9A4, 1968.
24. Stokes, K.B. (Personal Communication).
25. Salyer, I.O., Blardinelli, A.J., Ball, G.L. III, Weener, W.E., Gott, V.L., Ramos, M.D. and Furuse, A.: *J. Biomed. Mater. Res.* 1:105, 1971.
26. "Eccoamp Electrically Conductive Adhesives, Coatings and Casting Resins," Emerson and Cuming, Inc., Canton, Mass.
27. Redemske, R.F.: Semiconductor Measurement Technology: Reliability Technology for Cardiac Pacemakers II-A Workshop Report. USDC/NBS Special Pub. #400-42, p. 14, August 1977.
28. Ferreira, L.A.: Reliability Technology for Cardiac Pacemakers III, USDC/NBS Proc. Workshop III, p. 21, Oct. 1977.
29. Thompson, Noel P.: (Personal Communication).
30. Thomas, R.W.: Semiconductor Measurement Technology: Reliability Technology for Cardiac Pacemakers. NBS/FDA Workshop NBS #400-28, p. 12, June 1976.
31. Bangs, E.R.: Reliability Technology for Cardiac Pacemaker III, USDC/NBS Proc. Workshop III, p. 53, Oct. 1977.

32. Friauf, W.S.: *IEEE Natl. Telemetry Conf.,* p.34, 1969.
33. Gilman, B.: Reliability Technology for Cardiac Pacemakers III, USDC/NBS Proc. Workshop III, p. 43, Oct. 1977.
34. American Society for Testing and Materials, Philadelphia, PA.
35. Schafft, H.A.: Semiconductor Measurement Technology: Reliability Technology for Cardiac Pacemakers. NBS/FDA Workshop, NBS#400-28, p. 12, June 1976.
36. Ruthberg, S.: Semiconductor Measurement Technology: Reliability Technology for Cardiac Pacemakers. NBS/FDA Workshop NBS #400-28, p. 15, June 1976.

POLYETHYLENE ARTIFICIAL TENDONS

J.W. Hodge, Jr.

General Engineer

C.W.R. Wade, Ph.D.

Research Chemist

*US Army Medical Bioengineering Research and Development Laboratory
Fort Detrick
Frederick, Maryland 21701*

ABSTRACT

A number of synthetic materials were investigated as possible materials of construction during the development of artificial tendons. These materials include nylons, dacrons, linens, stainless steels, and polyethylenes fabricated into double-loop or porous tape type artificial tendons. The polyethylenes are the object of this investigation, which considers primarily the porous tape type artificial tendons.

The properties of strength, elastic recovery, porosity, and flexibility were evaluated and compared for each type of material. Polyethylene mesh, with pore sizes up to 500 microns square, had strengths of about 15kg. Elastic recovery was acceptable and flexion of the polyethylene artificial tendons in excess of 2 million flex cycles did not affect the mesh.

On comparison of the mechanical properties of the polyurethane artificial tendons with those of human tendon, it would appear that reasonable replication is possible. However, extensive clinical testing is required to determine ultimate behavior in the biological system.

The opinions or assertions contained herein are the private views of the authors and are not to be construed as official or as reflecting the views of the Department of the Army or the Department of Defense.

KEY WORDS

Artificial Tendons, Polyethylene, Internal Prosthetics, Biomedical Polymers.

INTRODUCTION

Surgical restoration of the normal functions of severed, damaged, or destroyed tendons has been attempted from a number of different approaches. Hunter, in 1965, presented evidence to show that a new tendon bed or sheath could be established, and that an autogenous tendon graft could be inserted into the new sheath and anastomosed to regain motor function [1]. This concept goes back to the work of Biesalski in 1910 [2]. Techniques of neosheath formation and natural tendon grafting continue to meet with some success, but there are injuries in which these approaches are not applicable and the only recourse is an artificial device [3].

Research and development on artificial tendons in this laboratory have been done in a number of progressive stages, leading to two basic types of artificial tendons [4]. Basically, the two types are the porous tape and the double-loop devices (Figure 1). The porous tape artificial tendons, consisting primarily of a porous tape surrounded by a medical grade silicone sheath, are designed to promote anastomosis through tissue ingrowth. The double-loop artificial tendons are designed for anastomosis of the device to tendon stumps by looping the residual natural tendon through the artificial tendon loop and suturing to itself. Also, both devices have a covering of medical grade silicone to isolate the basic construction materials from tissue and body fluids and to provide a smooth gliding surface when the artificial tendon is put in place.

The porous tape artificial tendons offer the advantage of anchoring by tissue ingrowth, and adjustable lengths from which shorter tendons can be made, depending on the surgical requirement. The double-loop artificial tendons are fabricated in fixed lengths but have the advantage of extra strength. While both artificial tendons have unique advantages, the clinical application seems to favor the porous tape artificial tendons. Tissue ingrowth into the pores of opening offered the best possibility for a sufficiently strong attachment between the artificial tendon and the remaining autogenous tendon. Consequently, the main thrust in this laboratory was shifted towards development of the porous tape devices.

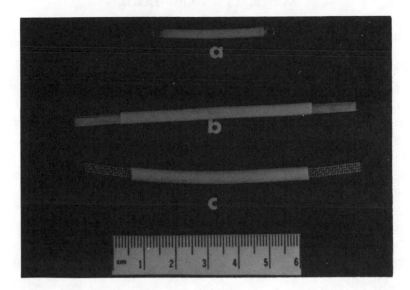

Figure 1. (a) Double loop tendon, (b) porous tape fabric mesh tendon, (c) porous woven tape tendon.

In addition to the types of artificial tendons, materials play a major and significant role in their design. Our selection of candidate materials for use in the development of the artificial tendons focused on reported requirements of tissue compatibility, in addition to the mechanical properties of strength, porosity, and flexibility [5]. During this effort, artificial tendons were fabricated from stainless steel wires, nylon (monofilaments), braided silk tapes, dacron tapes, and finally, polyethylene woven tapes and screens or meshes.

As expected, artificial tendons fabricated from fine stainless steel wires had very high strength properties but very poor flexibility. The stainless steel wires were abandoned early, primarily because of their failure under repeated flexing. Nylon monofilaments, although significantly more flexible than stainless steel wires, were rejected because their strengths were less than acceptable and there is evidence of their degradation in vivo. Dacron knitted tapes had sufficient strength and relatively high flexing ability, but under tension the change in the geometry of the pores had an adverse effect on tissue ingrowth. Because of these problems, polyethylene fabric meshes and woven tapes were selected as a structural material. In addition, these materials allowed for variation in pore sizes, flexibility, and provided adequate strength for this phase of study.

MATERIALS AND METHODS

Polyethylene Fabric Mesh and Woven Tapes

Fabric meshes and woven tapes of polyethylene were obtained from a commercial source (Prodesco Inc.). The fabric mesh materials contained uniform pores ranging in size from 111 microns square to 508 microns square. The mesh tapes were 0.5 mm to 1.0 mm in thickness and approximately 3 mm in width.

Polyethylene woven tapes contained pores in the 200 micron square range and were 0.5 mm in thickness and approximately 3 mm in width.

The mesh and woven tapes used in the fabrication of the artificial tendons (Figure 1, b and c) contained six or eight tension members (monofilaments) in parallel and side by side in the tape. Each monofilament in the six tension member structure was 0.2 mm in diameter. Each tension member in the eight tension member structure was 0.16 mm in diameter.

Silicone Outer Covering (Sheath)

Medical grade elastomer (382 Dow Corning) was mixed in accordance with the manufacturer's recommendations and placed in a special two-piece mold with a metallic core. The metal strip duplicated the size of the tapes which were 0.5 mm in thickness by 3.0 mm in width. After allowing for curing time, the silicone rubber tube was carefully removed from the mold and the metal strip was removed from the center silicone rubber, producing a sheath to cover the flat polyethylene tapes. The artificial tendon was formed by replacing the metal strip with the tapes which gave final devices 3.5-4 mm in width by 1.5 mm in thickness. The lengths were random but could be adjusted by cutting the devices to the length required for the surgical procedure.

Tensile Strength

Tensile strength was determined on a tension and compression test machine at a crosshead rate of 12.5 mm per minute. Elongation was determined as a function of jaw separation. A specimen approximately 8 centimeters in length was placed in serrated jaws and pulled at the specific rate. A gage length of 2.5 centimeters was the basic position from which the tension test started. A load-deformation curve was plotted from which the tensile strength was determined.

Ultimate stress was determined by dividing the break load by the combined cross-sectional area of all the tension members in the tape (6 or 8).

Pore Sizes

Pore sizes were determined by microscopic examination and measurement with a calibrated ocular. Pores in the fabric mesh tapes and the woven tape were generally rectangular in form as viewed under a 100× magnification.

Flex Test

Flexibility of the artificial tendons was determined by flexing or bending the specimen repeatedly through an angle of about 55°. One end of the artificial tendon was supported in a vise and the other end was attached through a spring to a reciprocating rod. As the reciprocating rod reached the end of its travel in both directions, the artificial tendon was loaded to approximately 2 kilograms. The equipment on which the test was conducted was operated at 60 cycles per minute. This amounted to 120 flexes per minute. The flex test involved a combination of bending and tension and essentially addressed durability under a load-flexing condition.

RESULTS AND DISCUSSION

Artificial tendons fabricated from a polyethylene fabric mesh containing six tension members (monofilaments), each 0.2 mm in diameter, produced an ultimate load of 15.4 kg (Table 1). This tensile strength is equal to 81.7 kg/mm². The fabric containing eight tension members, each 0.16 mm in diameter, produced an ultimate load of 7.8 kilograms which resulted in a tensile strength of 48.5 kg/mm². The elongation of both these devices was essentially the same at 65 and 66 percent, respectively. The woven tape withstood loads significantly less at 4.3 kg and a tensile strength of 22.8 kg/mm².

The stress-elongation properties (Figure 2) of these materials indicate that all the tape forms, while being polyethylene, do not behave the same under tension. This is probably the result of a particular post-treatment, a variation of the polymerization process, or more likely, the

Table 1. Properties of Polyethylene Artificial Tendon

Specimen	Tension Members	Ultimate Load (kg)	Tensile Strength (kg/mm^2)	Elongation (%)
Polyethylene Fabric Mesh (1)	6 (0.2 mm)	15.4	81.7	65
Polyethylene Fabric Mesh (2)	8 (0.16 mm)	7.8	48.5	66
Polyethylene Woven Tape	6 (0.2 mm)	4.3	22.8	68

(1) This polyethylene tape contained 6 parallel members in the longitudinal direction, each 0.20 mm in diameter.

(2) This polyethylene tape contained 8 parallel members in the longitudinal direction, each 0.16 mm in diameter.

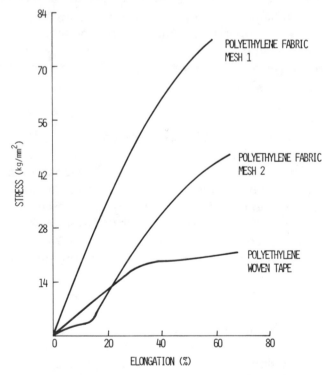

FIGURE 2. STRESS-ELONGATION CURVES OF POLYETHYLENE ARTIFICIAL TENDONS

geometric configuration of the structure itself. In any case, it would seem that the most important region of the stress-elongation curve would be that region in which the human tendon would fall. To replicate the tensile properties of human tendon, it was necessary to compare properties of these materials with the reported tensile properties of unembalmed human extensor tendom from a lower limb [6]. Analysis showed that the ultimate stress-strain values of the human tendon, which were 8.4 kg/mm^2 and 6 percent elongation, fell between polyethylene mesh 1 and the woven tape (Figure 3). While the tensile strength and ultimate elongation of the polyethylene materials are much greater than that of the human tendon, it does appear that the limits of the human tendon strength properties can be replicated with the polyethylene structures.

Reproduction of the strength properties of human tendon in an artificial equivalent appears to be a logical approach. Also, elastic recovery of the artificial device must be considered. The artificial tendon will experience some amount of deformation due to repetitive loading and unloading, but must be capable of regaining its original length to a great extent. It has been reported that calcaneal tendon has a 99 percent recovery just before rupture and immediately after removal of the stress [7]. For polyethylene tendons, with 10 percent elongation, there is a 70 percent elastic recovery immediately upon removal of the stress. The remaining 30 percent recovery is time dependent and occurs in a few minutes. If the polyethylenes were perfectly elastic materials, a 100 percent elastic recovery would have been immediately apparent on removing the stress. However, when the artificial polyethylene tendons are strained about 5 percent, there is an 80-90 percent elastic recovery. Again, the 10-20 percent elastic recovery remaining occurs in a short time (5 minutes). The 5 percent strain is acceptably near the working range of human tendon, which is reported to be about 3 percent [6].

Pore sizes determined from polyethylene fabric mesh materials similar to those used in the fabrication of the artificial tendons ranged from 111 microns square to 508 microns square. The pores were essentially square in appearance and the dimension given is the length of one side of the square. A 200 micron square pore diameter appears to be the size with the greatest potential for maximum strength through tissue ingrowth. Six polyethylene specimens having pore sizes of 111, 219, 286, 345, 436, and 508 microns square were evaluated. The diameter of the monofilaments from which the fabric mesh tapes were constructed varied considerably. Consequently, the strengths were similarly affected. The six specimens

Table 2. Pore Sizes and Break Loads of Polyethylene Fabric Mesh

Specimen	Pore Size (Microns Square)	Mean Break Load (kg)
1	111	3.75
2	219	4.94
3	286	8.35
4	345	8.39
5	436	9.75
6	508	12.43

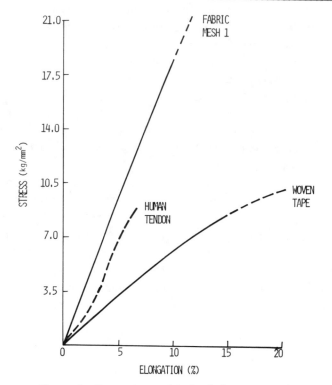

Figure 3. Comparison of Polyethylene Materials
and Human Tendon.

produced strengths of 3.74, 4.94, 8.35, 8.39, 9.75, and 12.43 kilograms, respectively, suggesting that artificial tendons with different strengths and porosities might be developed.

The flexibility of the polyethylene tendons appeared to be quite high, although there is no specific requirement for flexing of the artificial tendons. This is primarily due to the fact that there is no known number of flexes which the human tendon undergo. However, it was felt that the device should withstand at least 2 million flexes. Two specimens of the fabric mesh and woven tape artificial tendons were flexed in excess of 2 million times each without any apparent failures. Since the artificial tendons were loaded to approximately 2 kg during each flex, this test was a reasonably good indicator of flexibility as well as durability.

CONCLUSIONS

Polyethylene, one of a number of materials investigated, was fabricated into artificial tendons with variable strengths that could be selected according to the requirements of the surgical procedure. Also, the fabrication allowed for a selection of porosity. The choice of either of these characteristics and their combinations must ultimately be based on information developed through clinical and laboratory studies. This suggests that the next step in the development is the *in vivo* evaluation of these devices in chicken or other suitable models.

The ultimate utilization of these devices will depend on the ability to successfully attach them surgically with development of adequate strength through tissue ingrowth. The broad spectrum of pore sizes developed in this study should provide the necessary basis for initiating studies to determine the most desirable porosity for successful anastomosis.

The biocompatibility of the medical grade silicone (silastic) is well documented and was not a part of this study. However, polyethylene and other materials do not have the immense data in the biological systems, but the limited studies indicate its tissue reaction is minimal and may cause a mild response. Specific studies are necessary to completely determine biocompatibility.

In conclusion, the polyethylene tapes that were evaluated in this study appear to have sufficient strength, porosity, elastic recovery, and flexibility to fulfill the requirements of an artificial tendon, and replicate some of the properties of human tendon.

REFERENCES

1. Hunter, J.M.: *Artificial Tendons Early Development and Application.* Am. J. Surg., 109: pp. 325-338, 1965.
2. Biesalski, Konrad: *Veber Sehnenscheidenavswechslung.* Deutch Med. Wochnschur 36: pp. 1615-1618, 1910.
3. Hunter, J.M. and Salisbury, R.E.: *Flexor-Tendon Reconstruction in Severely Damaged Hands.* Jour. of Bone and Joint Surg., Vol. 53A, No. 5, pp. 829-858, 1971.
4. Wade, C.W.R., Ovellette, J.E., Hodge, J.W., Urban, J.J., and Salisbury, R.E., *Design and Fabrication of Two Types of Articial Tendons for Evaluation of Surgical Techniques,* J. Biomed. Mater. Res. Symposium, No. 6, pp. 149-155, 1975.
5. Lyman, D.J.: *Biomedical Polymers,* Biomaterials, Bement, A.L., Ed., Battelle Research Center, Univ. of Washington Press, pp. 269-283, 1971.
6. Benedict, J. Walker, L.B., Harris, E.H., *Stress-Strain Characteristics and Tensile Strength of Umembalmed Human Tendon.* J. Biomechanics 1: pp 53-63, 1968.
7. Yamada, H.: *Mechanical Properties of Locomotor Organs and Tissues:* Strength of Biological Materials, Evans, F.G., Editor, Baltimore, MD, Williams and Wilkins Co., pp. 99-101, 1970.

PERCUTANEOUS LEADS FOR ARTIFICIAL HEARTS AND OTHER PROSTHETIC DEVICES*

William J. Robinson

*Thermo Electron Corporation
Research and Development Center
Waltham, MA 02154*

and

Benedict D.T. Daly, Jr.

*Department of Cardiothoracic Surgery
Tufts New England Medical Center
and St. Elizabeth's Hospital
Boston, MA*

ABSTRACT

Support for patients in chronic organ failure often requires the use of long-term leads that traverse the skin for the conduction of fluids or electrical power. The extended use of support systems has been hampered by the lack of satisfactory percutaneous transmission systems. Problems of sepsis or inflammation at foreign body/tissue interfaces have remained major obstacles to be overcome in permanently implanted devices. These problems are compounded by the presence of axial loads, large diameter prostheses, and the mobility of the skin surface, which are unavoidable factors of systems intended for human use. Our laboratories are engaged in the development and testing of a percutaneous lead system that will interface with a human host for a minimum period of two years. The system addresses the characteristics of the human skin, the

*Supported, in part, by National Institutes of Health Contract NO1-HV-8-2919.

in vivo properties of certain synthetic polymers, the experience with various experimental and clinical transcutaneous conduits, and the systems with which they are used. This chapter describes the work to date and the resultant composite design.

KEY WORDS

Percutaneous leads, Epidermis, Dermis, Subcutaneous, Skin, Fibroblasts, Collagen, LVAD, Electrical Power, Vent line, Polytetrafluoroethylene, Polyurethane, Carbon coating (Biolite), Titanium alloy, Polyester velour, Nylon velour, Rubber, Silicone rubber, Abdominal wall, Miniature pigs.

INTRODUCTION

The extended use and evaluation of temporary and permanent left ventricular assist devices (LVAD's) and total artificial hearts has been hampered by the lack of satisfactory percutaneous energy transmission systems. Not unlike other applications, problems at the skin/prosthesis interfaces, in the form of sepsis or inflammation, and lack of attention to human requirements have remained as major obstacles to success. This chapter describes a Percutaneous Energy Transmission System (PETS) that addresses the biologic and engineering considerations associated with the use of percutaneous leads.

The design of a successful percutaneous lead system requires that the eventual prosthesis be compatible with the biologic characteristics of human tissues at the various biomaterial-tissue interfaces, as well as account for the mechanical forces and constraints imparted by such systems for extended periods of time, if not indefinitely. Our studies have examined carefully all of the biological characteristics of human skin and deeper tissues as well as the effect of available, compatible biomaterials at similar interfaces already in use. Armed with this information and considering the limitations or constraints imparted by support systems and the history of human behavior in relationship to other devices, a lead has been developed that fulfills the requirements of a successful PETS.

The system contains five major components, each serving a specialized purpose: (1) a flexible polyurethane conduit; (2) a carbon-coated titanium button at the epidermal level; (3) a porous polytetrafluoroethylene (PTFE) collar at the dermal and subdermal levels; (4) a semirigid polyurethane flanged skirt located in the subdermal subcutaneous tissue; and (5) a polyester velour covering that extends from the PTFE collar to the termination of the conduit. The carbon-coated button is relatively innocuous to the epidermis. The PTFE collar encourages collagen ingrowth and the subsequent inhibition of epidermal downgrowth. Polyester velour promotes rapid tissue ingrowth, thus providing a tenacious bonding in deeper tissues. Strain relief is imparted by the velour covered skirt, and the tunneling and velour covered conduit in deeper tissues.

In order to appreciate the need for a composite system, one must examine the systems with which it is to be used, the properties of human tissue and the results of previous investigations.

Artificial Heart Applications

In recent years, a great deal of attention has been focused on the development of temporary and permanent left ventricular assist device systems and total artificial hearts. Short of totally implanted systems (nuclear), a transcutaneous source of energy must be employed to supply these devices. For short-term use (up to two weeks), currently available percutaneous leads are satisfactory. Extended evaluation, however, has been hampered by problems of sepsis or inflammation originating at the foreign-body skin interface. Numerous approaches have been taken in recent years in an attempt to overcome problems associated with biomaterials traversing the skin for different applications. For some applications significant progress has been made and acceptable, though not ideal, techniques are currently employed. This is the case, for example, with dialysis shunts, hyperalimentation lines, and temporary electrodes. None of these systems, however, incorporates large (1 cm or greater) tubes or systems with significant mechanical stresses imparted at the skin interface.

Two types of leads can be considered for potential use in artificial heart systems: pneumatic and electrical. The size of pneumatic conduits depends on an acceptable compromise between engineering and physiologic considerations. Small lines are desirable from a physiologic viewpoint, whereas large lines are favored from a functional viewpoint to minimize fluid flow resistance, thus providing higher efficiency and better control. During pump systole, smaller diameter lines require more energy from the driver to displace a given volume of blood. During pump diastole, the smaller lines require higher physiologic pressures to fill the pump with blood. With an electrically driven LVAD, a pneumatic vent line is necessary to compensate for the piston displacement of the pulsatile pump. In this situation, a volume of air equivalent to the stroke volume must be moved through the vent line twice on each pump stroke cycle: air is vented to the atmosphere as the pump fills and is drawn inward as the pump ejects. Small lines could waste as much as 10 percent (0.6 watts loss/6 watts supplied) of the electrical power supplied to such a unit as indicated by Table 1, which shows the pressure drops and associated power losses for different sized vent lines on an LVAD system. Through a series of studies, it has been determined that vent tubing should not be less than 6.25 mm internal diameter. With necessary reinforcement and wall thickness, the resulting outside diameter would be 1 cm.

Table 1. Characteristics of an LVAD System, with Different Sized Vent Lines. Operating at 80 bpm, 75 ml Stroke Volume, and 250 ms Ejection Duration.

Vent Line Internal Diameter (mm)	Systolic Pressure Drop (mmHg)	Diastolic Pressure Drop (mmHg)	Combined Power Loss (watts)
3.5	32.0	17.0	0.60
4.0	24.0	9.0	0.38
4.5	17.0	3.0	0.18
5.0	9.0	2.0	0.10
5.5	5.5	1.3	0.07
6.0	3.0	1.0	0.05
6.5	2.2	0.8	0.03
7.0	1.4	0.6	0.02

Percutaneous cables for electrically actuated systems present different considerations than those of pneumatic conduits. Systems that are currently under development require multiple conductors. At least two conductors are required for power transmission and as many as eight conductors may be required for control and monitoring signals. Because of the current handling requirements, the power conductors are, of necessity, much larger wire gauges than the signal conductors and thus determine the ultimate size of the cable.

Electrical cables must be able to withstand constant flexing, be resilient enough to prevent erosion of adjacent soft tissue, and be chemically stable within the biologic environment. Although most in vivo experience has been with various neurologic stimulator conductors such as pacemaker leads, it is unlikely that the majority of this technology is directly applicable to LVAD systems because of the difference in energy levels between the two applications. Peak power levels of pacemaker systems are typically measured in milliwatts whereas the LVAD drive systems outputs are measured in watts, obviously several orders of magnitude higher. As a result, cable metals that are tolerated for neurologic applications because of their biologic compatibility (in spite of their relatively poor conductive properties) may not be usable in the LVAD systems. For example, the resistivity of platinum/irridium (PI), a common pacemaker electrode material, is over 15 times greater than that of copper. This means that for the same power dissipation, a PI conductor would have to be approximately 10 wire gauges larger than a comparable copper conductor. Copper presents a problem because it is highly reactive and corrodes easily when exposed to biologic liquids. Therefore, a copper conductor would have to be isolated both electrically and hermetically in a cable. In preliminary design studies, we have determined that copper conductors of size 25 AWG will meet the conduction requirements for a 12 volt system. With copper insulation, passivation, and strain relief, a cable will be approximately 4 mm in diameter. This is smaller than that required for pneumatic conduits and thus allows the use of smaller conduits for electrical cables.

Human Factors

The skin interface has received the most attention and is the major source of problems. Human skin provides several functions indispensible to life [1]. It protects against mechanical, thermal, chemical and radiant insults, participates in heat regulation via eccrine sweating and blood vessels and serves the nervous system with afferent stimulation. Skin is composed of three layers: epidermis, dermis, and subcutaneous tissue. Four adnexal or epidermal appendages give skin the remarkable ability to repair itself. These include the eccrine sweat glands, apocrine glands, hair follicles, and sebaceous glands. Skin in different regions differs vastly to adapt to special stresses. Langers lines are nonvisible cleavage planes in the skin. Their distribution has been mapped and their presence is a consideration in PETS placement.

The epidermis is a cellular membrane devoid of lymphatics, blood vessels, and significant amounts of connective tissue. It is parasitic on the dermis. Most epidermis contains two layers, the stratum malpighii and stratum corneum. The former consists of living cells and the latter dead cells from the former layer. Cells in the stratum malpighii originate from a basal layer. By division, daughter cells are produced which are displaced outward. These daughter cells and basal cells are called keratinocytes because they form keratin. They are connected by numerous prickles or rod-shaped thickenings of adjacent cell walls to which microscopic fibrils or tonofilaments (keratin precursor) are attached. Over the course of approximately 4 weeks these cells move toward the surface, progressively flattening as they move. They eventually shrink, lose their nuclei, and desquamate. The desquamating cells form the stratum corneum, a layer of interdigitated dead, flattened, cornified cells whose molecular framework is keratin — a tough fibrous protein. This latter layer is very hygroscopic and holds water avidly. During bathing, swelling and whitish wrinkling occurs; when dried, fissures and cracks develop exposing the underlying epidermis to physical and chemical trauma. Chronic inflammation results in increased mitotic activity in the epidermis and an increase in this outer layer.

From a practical point of view, the only skin appendages applicable are hair follicles, sebaceous glands, and the eccrine sweat glands. Each of these appendages located in the dermis can serve as a source of new cells for epidermal regeneration. The sebaceous glands are most abundant on the face, scalp, and scrotum. Normally they are only found in relation to hair follicles and secrete sebum — a complex lipoidal mixture. The eccrine sweat glands are more uniformly distributed and are composed of a duct opening in a free invisible pore and a secretory coil deep in the corium. Sweat is produced in response to sympathetic stimulation.

The corium or dermis is the major portion of skin and constitutes the most external of all connective tissue sheaths. Collagen fibers constitute the overwhelmingly predominant element. It is invaded by downgrowths of epidermis in the form of hair follicles and glands and contains an elaborate network of nerves, lymphatics, and blood vessels. Three cell types, all derivatives of the same primitive mesenchymal cell, are present — the fibrocyte, histiocyte, and mast cell. The fibrocyte or fibroblast produces collagen and small amounts of elastin. Collagen is a flexible soft protein with great resistance and tensile strength laid down as white branching fibers. Early immature collagen is called a reticulum fiber which matures by lateral association. Elastic fibers are single yellow fibers that branch and anastamose. Also present in the corium is a ground substance or matrix composed largely of mucopolysaccharides.

The subcutaneous tissue, composed primarily of fat, serves to protect and insulate, and acts as an energy source for the body. It is composed principally of lipocytes or fat cells. Its superficial layer contains the blood vessels and nerves that serve the overlying dermis.

Regeneration of damaged skin begins to take place almost immediately after any trauma. Even the peeling of cellulose tape off skin incites increased mitotic activity in the basal layer of the epidermis. When skin is injured, several processes begin to occur immediately. If the skin is penetrated, bleeding occurs from torn dermal capillaries concomitant with oozing from interstitial and intracellular fluids. A coagulum composed of fibrin, cells, cellular debris, and eventually bacteria, forms and hardens to form as eschar. Polymorphonuclear leukocytes invade the damaged surface beneath the eschar separating it from the visible tissue. At the same time, fibroblasts move to the area and begin laying down new collagen. New capillaries begin to develop and a clean granulating surface is formed. The epidermal cells at the wound margin and cells from the hair follicles or glands within the wound begin to divide. Under normal circumstances they migrate from the base to surface of skin in an upward direction, so to speak. When separated from their sister cells, they begin to more woundward seeking contact with another epidermal cell. This wanderlust is normally satisfied only when the cell has complete contact with other epidermal cells on all sides. Repletion of cells occurs through a chalone feedback system. Once the wound has been completely epithelialized, the granulating bed matures, and scar formation develops by contraction. Although the process of collagenization is complete at about 2 weeks, increases in wound tensile strength continue to occur for about 2 months.

When any foreign material is implanted transcutaneously, even a simple suture, the basic principles of skin regeneration continue to operate. Epithelial cells devoid of contiguity migrate in search of a sister cell. This migration takes the cells down along the path of the foreign material into the depths of the wound. This process is apparently inhibited by mature collagen. Thus contact inhibition occurs at the basal layer of the epidermis where cells sit on the basement membrane and underlying collagen.

In humans, one additional factor has to be considered: the skin is much more closely attached to the underlying tissues than that of many of the animals used in past experimentation. However, a certain mobility of the skin over subcutaneous tissues does exist. Further mobility is imparted by movement of the subcutaneous tissues over the fascia.

We believe that the preferable anatomic location for LVAD percutaneous leads in man is the anterolateral abdominal wall between the costal margin and the waistline. In this area, there is abundant soft tissue to relieve the strains imposed by percutaneous implants. In addition, this anatomic location provides several closely associated muscle layers ideal for tunnelling a device. We would place the exit site lateral to the rectus abdominis muscle. The system would penetrate the external and internal oblique fascia and muscles at right angles and would be tunnelled between the internal oblique and transversalis muscles to a blood pump or intracorporeal energy source either in the retroperitoneum or chest wall. This plane is rich in loose fibroconnective tissue with an excellent blood supply. It is also accessible to the patient from both a visual and manipulative point of view. In this location, it can be easily seen and cared for and, in addition, it is more accessible should repair or replacement be necessary.

Experience with Percutaneous Devices

The employment of various percutaneous leads in clinical and experimental settings has served mainly to emphasize the biologic nature of the skin. Certain principles have emerged which, when followed, permit degrees of symbiosis or tissue tolerance. In general, materials developed or used for percutaneous applications fall into one of three categories: smooth surfaced, rough textured, and porous. Each exhibits certain characteristics and the successful use of each varies in relationship to skin anatomy and physiology as well as a post-implantation hygiene and maintenance.

At the clinical level, arteriovenous shunts have been used for renal dialysis for several years [2,3]. These shunts are typically between an artery and its complementary vein and involve two percutaneous sites, one tube that originates at the artery and is connected externally to a second tube that returns to the vein. Initially these shunts were fabricated of polytetrafluoroethylene; most are now silicone rubber with polytetrafluoroethylene connectors. Many access routes have been used — the most common site is on the palmar surface of the forearm utilizing the radial or ulnar artery and the complementary vein. Arteriovenous shunts are examples of smooth surfaced percutaneous leads. Many shunts function for periods in excess of one year and as long as two years. Their remarkable success, however, has to be analyzed in the context of their utilization. By location and proper dressing between uses, they are essentially immobile, except during use. Furthermore, since the wound exist is in a state of controlled or local sepsis continuously, it is critical that these shunts have scrupulous care. The skin/biomaterial surface never joins as a unit and the epidermis grows inward creating a superficial sinus tract.

Percutaneous leads utilized for external pacemakers have had similar success for periods of up to 4 years [4]. Other examples include percutaneous electrodes occasionally supported with smooth buttons which have been successful for over 5 years [5]. Of the clinically utilized systems, several factors are apparent. No union occurs; all have superficial sinus tracts; all are relatively immobile; and all are small in size with diameters that are less than 3 mm.

In conjunction with circulatory support development, a number of large smooth surfaced buttons were designed for PETS [6,7]. All have had varying degrees of success and all have fared poorly once axial loads have been applied to them. [8]. Experience gleaned from these and other experiments has only served to emphasize that small — and large-diameter tubes, and immobile and mobile tubes, behave differently [9]. Using smooth tubes, completely strain-relieved percutaneous drivelines have survived for many months [10].

Rough textured materials for percutaneous leads have been investigated in many laboratories including our own [11,12,13]. Composites with polyester velour bonded to silicone rubber have been used successfully in LVAD experiments in calves for periods of up to 5 months duration over the past 5 years. The most successful system utilizes 1 cm outside diameter tubes with a compression spring for reinforcement. This arrangement evolved over time; the original tube was smooth rubber, 1.3 cm outside diameter. The evolution is shown in Table 2.

Certain findings have been demonstrated regarding the use of rough textured surfaces. Both nylon and polyester velour demonstrate rapid tissue ingrowth and excellent adhesion. Polyester is superior to nylon because it does not degrade over time. Coarse velour is better than fine velour. A series of biomaterial implants were performed in our laboratories to determine the adhesive strength of tissue to various materials and surface preparations. The results are shown in Table 3.

At the skin interface, rapid epidermal adherence occurs. However, two phenomena detract from its utilization at the skin surface. When the epithelium contacts the polyester velour it forms a tenacious mechanical-

Table 2. The Evolution of a Lead System that is Currently
Employed with Pneumatically Actuated LVAD Systems for both

Tubing	Covering	Skin Interface Results
Viton Rubber	None	Gross Septic Sinus Tract Formation
Viton Rubber	Nylon Velour Sleeve	Septic Sinus Tract Formation after few weeks
Silicone Rubber	Nylon Velour Sleeve	Septic Sinus Tract Formation after two months; Nylon degradation
Silicone Rubber	Bonded Polyester Flock	Septic Sinus Tract Formation after few weeks
Silicone Rubber	Polyester Velour Sleeve	Septic Sinus Tract Formation after few weeks
Silicone Rubber	Bonded Polyester Sleeve	Good ingrowth and seal; occasional local skin infection

Table 3. Adhesion Levels of Several Biomaterials. Studies were
Conducted with Test Pieces (1 cm × 5 cm) Implanted in the Subcutaneous Abdominal Fascia of Adult Rabbits. Measurements
are in g/cm.

Materials and Surface	High	Low	Mean	S.D.
Polyester Velour #6000K 61121, Coarse with Silastic Back	>500	152.6	373.1	143.8
Polyester Velour #6107, Fine with Silastic Back	>333	87.5	201.4	96.7
Salt Leached Texture Tecoflex HR	63.7	6.5	24.7	21.0
Integral Flock Tecoflex HR	31.4	0	14.0	16.4
500μ Flocked Tecoflex HR	26.7	13.3	20.8	4.4
250μ Flocked Tecoflex HR	16.5	11.6	13.7	2.5
Smooth Tecoflex HR	0	0	0	0
Biomer, Smooth	0	0	0	0
LTI Carbon Discs, Smooth	0	0	0	0

chemical bond which satisfies its desire to migrate. However, as these
cells now continue the normal maturation process, they pull the velour
toward the surface. This is an experimental observation not confirmed in
humans. Polyester velour-covered drivelines have been used to power
left ventricular assist devices in both man and animals. In man, the duration has been short. In animals, continual stress at the skin interface produces epithelial detachment, tissue trauma, and eventually infection.

In a series of velour-lined prosthesis experiments by Pae, et al., the principle of immobilization was again employed [14]. Utilization of both a skirt in the subcutaneous tissue and an extracutaneous flange substantially improved results.

Of the porous materials; i.e., materials which have pores of sufficient magnitude to allow tissue ingrowth, we have been most impressed with the results of Winter utilizing polytetrafluoroethylene porous membrane (Porous PTFE) [15]. In comparison with other porous materials, films, and sponges, porous PTFE implants caused the epidermis to form a stable ring of tissue about the implants near the skin surface with little tendency to growing down into dermis. At 15 days this ring of tissue was located 1 mm below the skin surface. The pores allowed blood vessels and connective tissue cells to invade the material forming fibrous tissues which provided the biologic basis for inhibiting epidermal migration.

Pets Design Rationale

In designing a PETS, we have closely examined the physiology of skin maturation and the reaction of various materials to this process, keeping in mind that man is the intended recipient. Human experience with available systems and the restraints imparted by the PETS were factors in design. We do not believe that a single material exists at the present time that has a uniform consistency and structure and that would be accepted and incorporated by human tissue at the skin level and in deep tissues. We do believe, however, that a composite lead can specifically interface with the biologic characteristics at each level and account for the mechanical forces and constraints imparted by PETS.

The basic tube will serve as a conduit for electric, pneumatic, or hydraulic systems allowing for the incorporation of special hardware within its lumen as each specific system dictates. The PETS has five major components, each serving a specialized purpose. The basic conduit is polyurethane 1 cm in outer diameter. Polyurethane was chosen because it is relatively inert, is sufficiently strong to withstand the pneumatic or hydraulic pressures necessary to drive blood pumps over significant periods of time (in excess of 2 years), and is also flexible. This flexibility reduces stresses at prosthesis-tissue interfaces. It is also a basic component of drivelines currently used in experimental and clinical systems.

External to the polyurethane tube are four major components: a carbon coated button at the epidermal level; a porous PTFE interface at the dermal and subdermal level; a subdermal subcutaneous polyurethane skirt, rigid but flexible and overcoated for 1 cm adjacent to the tube with porous PTFE and the remainder of the top and bottom coated with polyester velour; and the remaining portion of the tube is covered with polyester velour bonded with strippable adhesive.

Smooth carbon was chosen to be the epidermal interface. We believe it is impossible to eliminate shear forces at the epidermal level with a 1 cm tube connected to an external unit. The human body is not a rigid structure and no reasonable site for the unit exists that would be completely devoid of some motion. Shear forces disrupt tissue ingrowth into either velour or porous materials and produce microhemorrhage, tissue exudation, or necrotic cellular debris that serve as nidi for infection [16]. The carbon with a smooth nonporous nonreactive surface allows the surface epithelium to grow to the device and down along its neck. As the cells grow downward they become modified and nondesquamating, producing a dry sinus tract. Meticulous care to this wound site allows for a clean sinus. The same wound management that dialysis patients receive is utilized at this level. The carbon button is flanged externally. Flanges have been demonstrated to strain relieve percutaneous tubes at the skin surface [14].

Beneath the carbon is short vertical segment of porous PTFE extending partially out over a skirt. The porous PTFE provides a transition material allowing blood vessel and fibroblast invasion with collagen production. This collagen barrier provides the feedback inhibition necessary to interface with downgrowing epidermal cells permitting a stable epidermal ring to form. Although tissue bonding to PTFE undoubtedly is not strong we have strategically placed it at a position on the PETS where there is relatively little shear stress.

In order to eliminate the natural gliding of skin over subcutaneous tissue, a 5 cm diameter polyurethane flanged skirt is used. The ring is rigid radially but flexible axially. Any shear at the tube exit, or motion in the region of exit, is distributed over a relatively broad area. All but about the first centimeter is overcoated with polyester velour to promote the rapid ingrowth of fibroconnective tissue to provide strong adherence. The skirt is positioned in the subcutaneous plane subadjacent to the subcutaneous tissue carrying the dermal blood supply, lymphatics and nerves. In addition, the skirt contains six holes that allow tissue ingrowth and lymphatic drainage.

The remaining portion of the conduit is covered with polyester velour to promote the rapid ingrowth of fibroconnective tissue. This portion of the tube provides internal stability and is tunnelled through muscular layers. The polyester velour, however, is bonded to the polyurethane in a manner permitting its detachment should a clinical situation warrant transplantation of the PETS to a different site. In such a situation a conduit terminal (carbon, porous PTFE, and skirt section of the tube) could be mated to the deeper polyurethane tube using a connector and sleeve and the deeper tube would then be rebonded to polyester velour.

While a composite design makes a PETS somewhat complex, it must be remembered that several totally different biologic tissues are being traversed we believe this conduct accounts for the characteristics of the transversed tissues and the materials selected in addition to meeting the strain relief at both the skin surface with the flange and the subcutaneous tissue-dermal interface with the skirt and, in the deeper tissues, with polyester velour and a tunnelling procedure. The carbon minimizes tissue reaction and, hence, inflammation at the skin surface; the porous PTFE develops a collagenous collar to inhibit epithelial downgrowth; and polyester velour permits the rapid development of tissue adhesiveness to stabilize the system.

Design and Fabrication

The program goals included the design and fabrication of a practical PETS system that could be tested in our animal model and then be translated easily into an LVAD system intended for use in the human. In essence, this approach has been followed, and a basic design was established and is being successfully tested.

Several materials are used in this composite design: (1) titanium alloy button; (2) smooth carbon coating; (3) porous polytetrafluoroethylene (PTFE); (4) special polymer adhesive for bonding PTFE; (5) semirigid polyurethane disc; (6) strippable polymer adhesive; (7) flexible polyurethane tubing; and (8) polyester velour. Each material has been chosen for a particular function. The tissue contacting surfaces are smooth carbon, porous PTFE and polyester velour. Figure 1 shows a detailed view of the top section of the prosthesis.

The base portion of the skin button is titanium alloy, Ti-6Al-4V. The crown portion of this button is coated with biocompatible glassy carbon deposition, Biolite, by General Atomic in San Diego. Biolite has the same biological properties as pyrolytic carbon, but is not as hard; however,

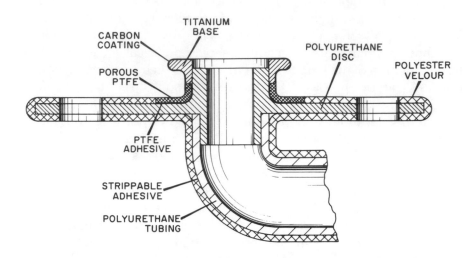

Figure 1. Detailed view of the cutaneous (top) section of the PETS.

hardness is not a requirement for this application. As illustrated, only the tissue-contacting surface is carbon coated. The buttons are machined from rods, polished, and inspected. After passing inspection, they are shipped to General Atomic for Biolite coating.

The porous polytetrafluoroethylene (PTFE) is the same type that is used as vascular graft, Gore-tex. Gore-tex is acquired in its vascular graft form in 35 cm lengths. The graft material is divided longitudinally and flattened to form a long sheet; discs are die cut from the sheet, formed over a fixture and bonded to the semirigid polyurethane disc.

Coarse polyester velour is used for deep tissue anchoring. Velour is obtained in sheet form. Sections cut from the sheet are formed over the PETS structural pieces, the disc and tubing, and bonded in place.

The remaining constituents are polyurethane. A family of biocompatible urethanes has been developed in our laboratories for use in biomedical prostheses. With slight modifications in formulation, these materials can be used as rigid parts, semirigid pieces, or soft components. All of the monomers have been chosen to permit 100 percent reactive curing, which results in finished polymers that will not leach plasticizers or other potentially irritating substances.

The polyurethane disc that serves as the structural component of the subcutaneous skirt is a semirigid material, which is bendable to absorb forces normal to the tissue surface but is rigid radially to restrain motion across the surface. The porous PTFE and polyester velour are bonded to this piece using polyurethane adhesives. The PETS disc is machined from a molded thick disc of a two-component reactive mixture of 100 percent solids. Figure 2 presents the molecular composition of the rigid elastoplastic. This is a highly crosslinked polyurethane synthesized from hydrogenated methylene diisocyanate (HMDI) and an ethylene oxide-capped trimethylol propane (ETMP) crosslinker. The high degree of crosslinking imparted by the ETMP produces a longitudinal flexibility, characteristics that are ideal for this application.

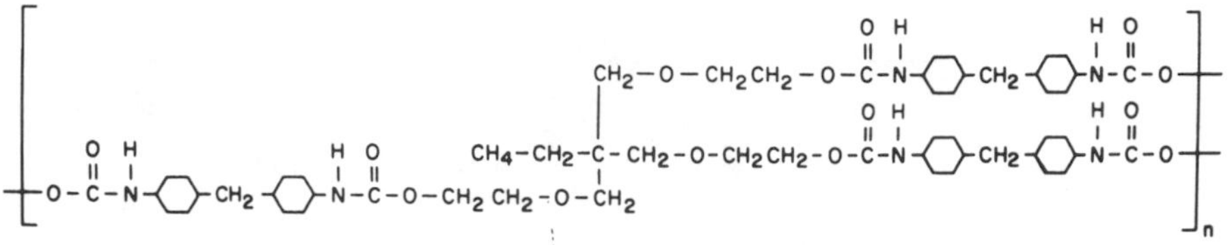

Figure 2. Molecular architecture of rigid elastoplastic.

The tubing is a flexible polyurethane synthesized from a linear segmented elastomer derived from HMDI, a 2000 molecular weight polytetramethylene ether glycol (PTMEG), and butanediol (BD). Figure 3 shows the structural architecture of this flexible polyurethane.

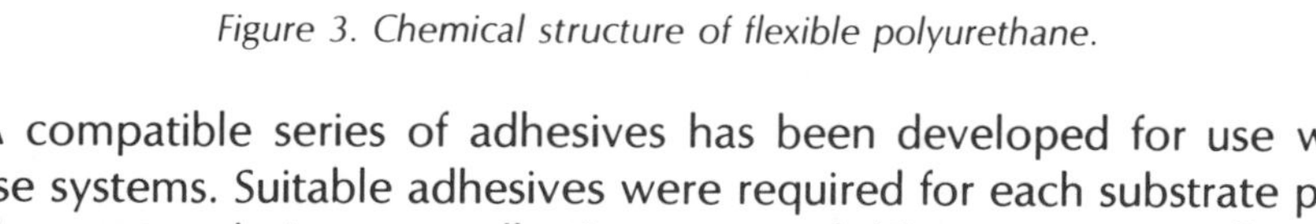

Figure 3. Chemical structure of flexible polyurethane.

A compatible series of adhesives has been developed for use with these systems. Suitable adhesives were required for each substrate pair. In the present design, two adhesives are used: (1) a permanent adhesive; and (2) a strippable adhesive. The permanent adhesive is used for all joints except the polyester velour to polyurethanes; the adhesive used at the polyester velour joints is a pressure-sensitive elastomer intended to be strippable to accommodate the possible removal and insertion of a new PETS postimplant.

The permanent adhesive required a special formulation to be developed to ensure adhesion of the porous PTFE to the polyurethane disc. The resulting adhesive is based on a 1/1/1 stoichiometric ratio of HMDI, polybutadiene glycol and N,N'-bis (2-hydroxypropyl) aniline. The resulting structure of the reactants is highly complex; for simplicity, the molecular structures of the monomers used in this adhesive are presented in Figure 4. During cure, all hydroxyl groups react with the iso-cyanate moities, resulting in urethane linkages.

CHEMICAL NAME	CHEMICAL STRUCTURE
Hydrogenated MDI	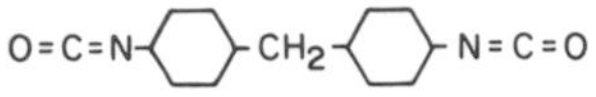 $O=C=N-\langle\ \rangle-CH_2-\langle\ \rangle-N=C=O$

Polybutadiene
  trans 1,4 60%
  cis 1,4 20%
  vinyl 1,2 20%
	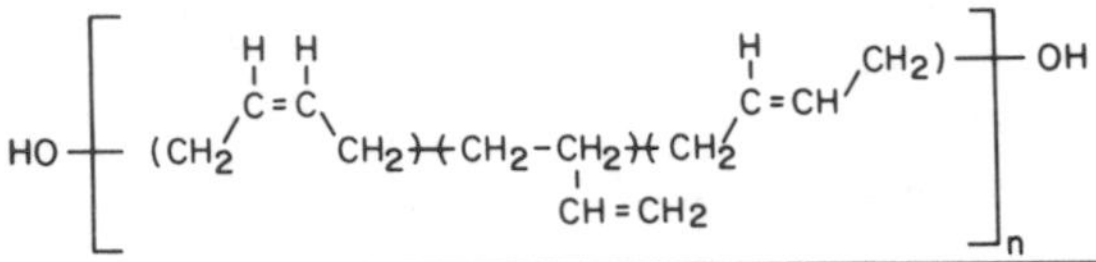

$N_1 N^1$ bis $\left[\,2\text{ hydroxypropyl}\,\right]$ aniline	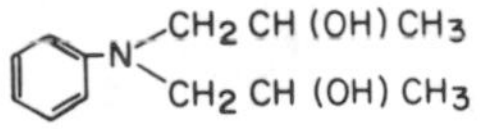

Figure 4. Reactive monomers utilized in PTFE adhesive.

The strippable adhesive is based on a quick-crystallizing elastomer, synthesized from methylene diisocyanate (MDI), polycaprolactone glycol (PCL), and butanediol (BD). The chemical structure of the cured polymer is shown in Figure 5. The adhesive is fabricated by dissolving this cured

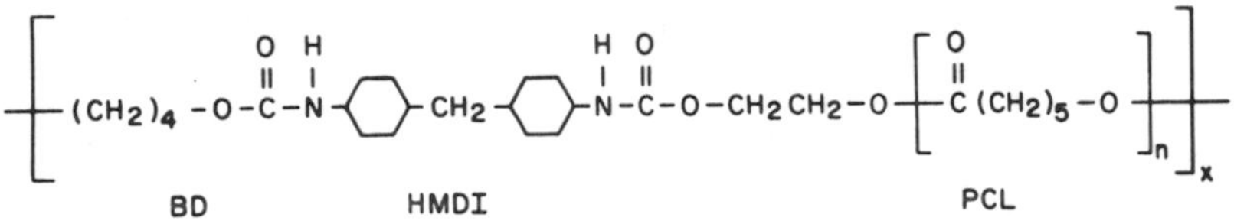

Figure 5. Chemical structure of quick-crystallizing elastomer.

polyurethane in a mixture of methyl ethyl ketone and tetrahydrofuran, 10 percent nonvolatiles; a small quantity (1.0 percent by weight) of a soft vinyl resin is added to serve as a tackifying resin. The degree of adherence of the strippable adhesive is a compromise between the force required to peel the polyester velour from the polyurethane tubing and the functional adherence between the velour and connective tissue. Polyester velour was chosen for this application because it promotes rapid ingrowth of connective tissue which results in a tenacious bond between the velour and the tissue. The peel strength of the tissue/velour bond is approximately 150 g/cm. The strippable adhesive had to have at least that much adhesion to the tubing so that the tissue would not gradually pull the velour from the tubing. Therefore, a safety factor in adhesive strength was one of the developmental criteria for this adhesive. The design point of the formula strippable adhesive is aimed at a bonding strength of approximately 300g/cm, or twice that of the tissue/velour bond, permitting the velour to be removed from the tube if necessary, for repair of the conduit at some time postimplant. The longterm properties of the adhesive have yet to be examined, however, so no definitive results can be presented at this time.

Fabrication Procedures

The fabrication of the PETS systems requires the combination of several discrete materials. The initial preparation of each material is conducted in a separate and distinct fashion from that of any other material. Each material is then joined into the system in a sequential manner. A simplified flow chart is presented in Figure 6 to show the fabrication process. This chart excludes many of the specific fabrication, testing, and cleaning steps. Each step in the process is followed by appropriate quality control procedures.

The design and fabrication methods currently being utilized resulted from careful review and deliberation by the program staff. The intent was to arrive at a system that could be evaluated in the most meaningful manner. For example, the original concept called for adhesively bonding the titanium alloy button to the polyurethane conduit. This would have resulted in a great degree of difficulty when the prosthesis was to be sectioned for histologic samples and would have probably distorted the soft tissues in the areas of the button. It was decided, therefore, to provide a removable button. This is accomplished in the current design by providing a screw that holds the button in place. In situ, the screw also joins the button in compression with the porous PTFE.

High modulus polyurethane is cured in forms that approximate the diameter and overall height of the subcutaneous semirigid disc. The piece is machined into the desired shape and the center is drilled and

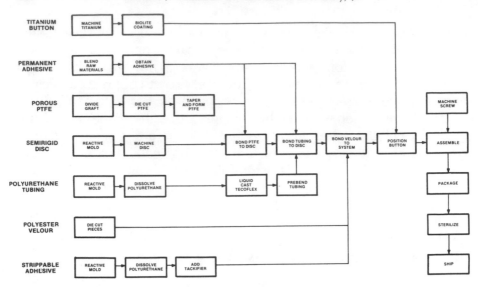

Figure 6. Flow chart for fabrication of PETS.

tapped. This semirigid disc provides the main frame for the PETS system; that is, it is the piece upon which all other parts of the composite are attached.

Titanium alloy is received as bar stock. The titanium buttons are then machined from the bar and polished in accordance with the standard procedures of our fabrication department. The buttons are inspected and tolerances are checked. Following inspection, the buttons are Biolite carbon coated. The buttons are put on the PETS as one of the last fabrication steps.

As mentioned, the porous PTFE is purchased in the form of vascular grafts. The porous surface of this material is shown in Figure 7. To use the PTFE in the PETS prosthesis, the PTFE must be first cut into the form of a disc, which is accomplished after the graft is divided longitudinally. The disc is then placed into a specially designed fixture to form the vertical collar of the PTFE section. The vertical collar is formed by using a two-piece fixture with male and female halves. The male half is shaped like the desired form of the PTFE while the female half is a receiver that has the inverse shape. The PTFE is placed on the female half and the vertical collar is formed as the male section gradually is worked so that the PTFE is carefully stretched into the female receiving section of the fixture. Care must be taken during this manipulation to maintain the integrity of the

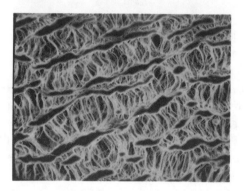

Figure 7. Scanning electron micrographs of PTFE porous surface: note that pores are tubular and loosely fibrillar.

PTFE porous surface. After being formed, the PTFE is bonded to the semirigid disc.

Tecoflex HR polyurethane is used for the subcutaneous conduit. A cured sheet of the urethane is made into a solution by dissolving the Tecoflex in dimethylacetamide. The solution is used for dip casting 15 cm tubes on a multiple mandrel mold. Following demolding, the tubes are placed on a special mandrel forming a curve in the end of the tube that attaches to the subcutaneous disc. This is done in a heat forming process by exposing the tubing and mandrel to 90°C dry heat for one hour.

After the PTFE is formed in the mold, the male half of the mold is removed. The permanent adhesive is applied to the PTFE and the semirigid disc is positioned where the male section was originally. The Tecoflex tube is bonded to the underside of the disc. Polyester velour pieces are cut with dies and the pieces are bonded to the uncovered portions of the disc and the outer walls of the tubing using the strippable adhesive. After the PTFE is bonded to the semirigid disc, the center hole of the disc is covered by the PTFE; the PTFE covering this hole is excised carefully so as not to disturb the remaining porous surface. The disc is perforated with six holes, 4 mm in diameter. The prosthesis is then cleaned by ultrasonication in deionized water for 30 minutes. The prosthesis is placed in its shipping fixture and dried at 45°C for 1 hour. The titanium button is positioned and secured with a ¼-20 screw to the semirigid disc.

RESULTS

Testing of the PETS conduit has been carried out in the miniature pig, which was chosen as an experimental model because of the similarity of its skin composition to that of man. Although some dimensional changes have resulted from attempts to optimize the prosthesis for use in the animal model, the basic design has remained essentially unchanged. All implants have appeared clinically satisfactory at explantation; gross and histopathologic results have varied somewhat with the different iterations. However, each of the initial hypotheses has been confirmed.

In a similar fashion to smooth surfaced conduits, a sinus tract forms; in contrast to the type of sinus formed with smooth prostheses, the PETS sinus tract is superficial and dry [17]. Typically, the sinus is lined with epidermal cells terminating at the porous PTFE collar. The appearance of the epidermal layer differs depending on the material in contact with it. When in contact with the PTFE, the cell layer is thin, only a few cells thick. Several of the skin buttons have been fabricated of titanium alloy alone, without the Biolite carbon coating; the epidermis in contact with these buttons is thickened and irregular — hyperkeratotic, acanthotic, and pappilomatose. In contrast, epidermis in contact with the Biolite surface is thicker than the normal, superficial epidermal layer, but tapers in a regular manner to the thin epidermal layer that forms a seal at the PTFE.

The pores of the PTFE permit fluid and cellular infiltration and subsequent collagen deposition by the fibroblasts within the material. The cellular infiltration and the collagen fibrillar detail within the PTFE architecture have been confirmed by electron microscopy [18]. This tissue ingrowth into the PTFE forms a stable bond which inhibits epidermal downgrowth permitting a tight epidermal/PTFE junction at the base of the sinus.

The polyester velour, which covers the subcutaneous skirt and intracorporeal portions of the conduit, forms a tenacious bond with all of the tissues in contact with it at the subcutaneous and muscular levels. The tissue reaction is characteristically that of a foreign body. In those animals in which the skirt was situated in the deep hypodermis or below it, insufficient skin immobility was achieved and deep sinus tract formation to the velour on the top of the skirt occurred. Because of the relatively weak tensile strength of the tissue/PTFE bond, immobilization by a subdermal or superficial subcutaneous skirt is essential for the maturation and longevity of a percutaneous lead. The inflammatory reaction produced by the polyester velour in the subcutaneous results in significant swelling of the tissue above the skirt in the first few days following implantation (maximum, 2 weeks); this swelling can be accommodated by providing adequate clearance between the flange and the skin button and the subcutaneous skirt.

CONCLUSION

In developing a percutaneous lead, it is necessary to understand the requirements of the application and then adapt the design to that application. The PETS described in this chapter utilizes a composite design and functions in symbiotic balance with the tissues it traverses. Experiments in our animal model have demonstrated a superficial sinus tract lined by epidermal cells. The tract terminates at a collagen barrier formed by the infiltration of the biologic constituents into the pores of the PTFE. The necessity of immobilization of the skin has been confirmed, being achieved by a subdermal, radially rigid skirt. The tenacious bonding of the prosthesis due to tunnelling through, and polyester velour interfaces in deep tissues provides the internal support required.

Although the application for the current development requires relatively large leads, the principles and basic design can be readily adapted to other applications such as arteriovenous shunts, hyperalimentation lines, and neurological leads. In those areas where the skin must be traversed for long time periods and where the possibility of infection is a severely limiting function, a lead that is able to adapt to the various tissue levels can be a significant help in reducing morbidity and extending the life expectancy of the affected patients.

REFERENCES

1.   Bloom, W. and Fawcett, D.W., *A Textbook of Histology*, 10th Edition, 23:563-597, W.B. Sanders, Philadelphia, 1975.

2.   Quinton, W., Dillard, D., and Scribner, B.H., Cannulation of Blood Vessels for Prolonged Hemodialysis, Trans. Amer. Soc. Artif. Intern. Organs, 6:104, 1960.

3.   Baily, G.L., Hampers, C.L., and Merrill, J.P., Home Hemodialysis: A Look Five Years Later, J. Amer. Med. Assoc., 212:1850, 1970.

4.   Schmedel, J.B. and Escher, D.J.W., Transvenous Electrical Stimulation of the Heart: 1. Cardiac Pacemakers, Annals of the New York Academy of Sciences III, 3:972, 1964.

5.   Mladejovsky, M.G., Eddington, D.K., Dobell, W.H. and Brackman, D.E., Artificial Hearing for the Deaf by Chochlear Stimulation: Pitch Modulation and Some Parametric Thresholds, Trans. Amer. Soc. Artif. Int. Organs, 2:1, 1975.

6.   Klain, M., and Nose, Y., Use of Laboratory Animals in Artificial Organs Research, Chapter 3, *Methods of Animal Experimentation*, Vol. 5, W.I., Ed., Academic Press, New York, 340-341, 1974.

7.   Nose, Y., Russell, F., Gradel, F., and Kantrowitz, A., Long-Term Operation of an Electronically Controlled Plastic Auxiliary Ventricle in Conscious Dog., Trans. Am. Soc. Art. Int. Organs, 10:140, 1964.

8.   Nose, Y., Discussion of Pae, W., Jr., et al.: Design and Evaluation of a Percutaneous Transthroacic Cannula, Trans. Am. Soc. Artif. Int. Organs, 22:142, 1976.

9.   Rawson, R.O., and Vasko, K.A., A Chronic Percutaneous Lead System Employing a Skin-Prosthesis Graft, J. Surg. Res., 8:274, 1968.

10. Kolff, W.J. and Lawson, J., Status of Artificial Heart and Cardiac Assist Devices in the United States, Trans. Amer. Soc. Artif. Int. Organs, 21:620, 1975.

11. Hall, C.W. and Ghidoni, J.J., Skin Interfacing Techniques, *Polymers in Medicine and Surgery*, R.L. Kronenthal, Ed., Plenum Press, New York, 167, 1974.

12. Keiser, J.T., Norman, J.C., and Bernhard, W.F., Pre-Clinical Evaluation of Temporary Assist Pumping, Thermo Electron Report No. NHLBI-NO1-HL-73-2946-2, 1975. Available from National Technical Information Service, Springfield, VA.

13. Keiser, J.T. and Poirier, V.L., Clinical Evaluation of Temporary Assist Pumping, Thermo Electron Report No. NHLBI-NO1-HV-5-3008-1, 1976. Available from National Technical Information Service, Springfield, VA.

14. Pae, W., Jr., O'Banion, W., Prophet, G.A., Donachy, J.H., Abt, A., and Pearce, W.S., Design and Evaluation of a Percutaneous Transthoracic Cannula, Trans. Amer. Soc. Artif. Intern. Organs, 22:135, 1976.

15. Winter, G.D., Transcutaneous Implants, Reaction of the Skin-Implant Interface, J. Biomed. Mat. Res. Symp., Vol. 5 (Part 1): 96, 1974.

16. Mooney, V. and Roth, A.M., Advances in Percutaneous Electrode Systems, Biomat. Med. Dev. ARt. Org., 4:171, 1976.

17. Szycher, M., Daly, B.D.T., Robinson, W.J. Keiser, J.T., and Haudenschild, C.C., Development of a Percutaneous Energy Transmission System, Proc. 7th New Eng. Bioeng. Conf., Troy, NY, 381-387, 1979.

18. Daly, B.D.T., et al., Development of Percutaneous Energy Transmission Systems, Annual Report No. NHLBI-NO1-HV-8-2919-1, 1979. Available from National Technical Information Service, Springfield, VA.

SUBJECT INDEX

AUTHOR INDEX

620/192 dan

547.7044/KOE